Statistical Epidemiology

We dedicate this book to Nicki and Asiyah.

Statistical Epidemiology

Graham R. Law[1] and Shane W. Pascoe[2]

[1]*Faculty of Medicine and Health University of Leeds, UK*
[2]*Pascoe Psychology Pty Ltd, New South Wales, Australia; and Centre for Primary Health Care and Equity, University of New South Wales, Australia*

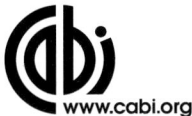
www.cabi.org

CABI is a trading name of CAB International

CABI
Nosworthy Way
Wallingford
Oxfordshire OX10 8DE
UK
Tel: +44 (0)1491 832111
Fax: +44 (0)1491 833508
E-mail: info@cabi.org
Website: www.cabi.org

CABI
38 Chauncey Street
Suite 1002
Boston, MA 02111
USA
Tel: +1 800 552 3083 (toll free)
Tel: +1 (0)617 395 4051
E-mail: cabi-nao@cabi.org

A catalogue record for this book is available from the British Library, London, UK.

Library of Congress Cataloging-in-Publication Data

Law, Graham R.
    Statistical epidemiology / Graham R. Law and Shane W. Pascoe.
        p. ; cm.
    Includes bibliographical references and index.
    ISBN 978-1-84593-816-1 (hb : alk. paper) -- ISBN 978-1-84593-796-6 (pbk. : alk. paper)
    I. Pascoe, Shane W. II. C.A.B. International. III. Title.
    [DNLM: 1. Epidemiologic Methods. 2. Epidemiologic Factors. WA 950]

614.4072'7--dc23

                                    2012036035

ISBN-13: 978 1 84593 816 1
ISBN-13: 978 1 84593 796 6

Commissioning editor: Rachel Cutts
Editorial assistant: Christopher Shire
Production editors: Fiona Chippendale and Shankari Wilford

Typeset by SPi, Pondicherry, India
Printed and bound by Gutenberg Press Limited, Tarxien, Malta

Contents

Mathematical and statistical symbols   vii

Preface   ix

1   Foundations of Epidemiology   1
    1.1   An Introduction   1
    1.2   Science and Its Methods   7
    1.3   The Importance of Epidemiology   14
    1.4   Samples and Populations   19
    1.5   Observational and Experimental Studies   25
    1.6   A Medical Sociological View   30

2   Cause and Effect   36
    2.1   The Meaning of Causation   36
    2.2   Models of Causation   42
    2.3   Visualizing Cause   47

3   An Epidemiologist's Toolkit   52
    3.1   A Problem for Epidemiology   52
    3.2   Anecdote   54
    3.3   Case Report, Case Series   59
    3.4   Cross-Sectional Survey   64
    3.5   Disease Registers and the Ecological Study   68
    3.6   Case-Control Study   75
    3.7   Cohort Study   83
    3.8   Randomized Controlled Trials   91
    3.9   Qualitative Research   102
    3.10   A Hierarchy of Evidence   108
    3.11   Systematic Review and Meta-Analysis   113
    3.12   An Answer From Epidemiology   117

4   Dealing With the Numbers   121
    4.1   Types of Data   121
    4.2   Presenting Data   125
    4.3   Measures of Location   131
    4.4   Measures of Spread   136
    4.5   Prevalence of Disease   139
    4.6   Incidence of Disease   143
    4.7   Risk of Disease   150
    4.8   Odds and Odds Ratios   158
    4.9   Hypothesis Testing   163
    4.10   Confidence Intervals   168

5   What Can Go Wrong: Error, Bias and Confounding   **173**

    5.1   Types of Error and Bias   173

    5.2   Information Bias   182

    5.3   Selection Bias   188

    5.4   Confounding   193

Answers and Feedback   **199**

References   **211**

Index   **217**

Mathematical and statistical symbols

AR	Absolute risk
ARR	Absolute risk reduction
c_1	Number captured on 1st list (capture-recapture)
c_2	Number captured on 2nd list (capture-recapture)
e_0	Number of exposed controls or non-cases
e_1	Number of exposed cases
e_{as}	Expected number of cases in strata a and s
EER	Exposed event rate
$f(x)$	Function of x
i	An index for a variable
I	Incidence rate
ITT	Intention-to-treat analysis
IQR	Inter-quartile range
n	Number of values in sample or population
n_1	Number of cases
n_t	Number in population during time period t
n_{as}	Number in population in strata a and s
NNT	Number needed to treat
o_t	Number of observed new cases during time period t
OR	Odds ratio
P	Prevalence, point prevalence
$Q1$	Lower quartile of data
$Q3$	Upper quartile of data
r	Number recaptured on 2nd list (capture-recapture)
RR	Risk ratio
RRR	Relative risk reduction
SD	Standard deviation
SIR	Standardized incidence ratio
t	Time period
u_0	Number of unexposed controls or non-cases
u_1	Number of unexposed cases
UER	Unexposed event rate
w_i	Weighting variable for value i
x_i	Value i of a variable x
$\bar{x}$	Mean of values of x
$\bar{x}'$	Weighted mean of values of x

Preface

This book has been designed to form one of the core texts for undergraduate and postgraduate foundation courses in epidemiology and medical statistics. We provide a resource that will enable teachers and lecturers to build their course to teach their students core statistical epidemiology. Real examples are used to illustrate the concepts, covering many of the ground-breaking and pioneering epidemiological studies. All teachers, educators, trainers and facilitators of epidemiology and medical statistics may find this a useful resource book for pedagogic development.

The book is organized into bite-size sections. Each section can be considered as a reusable learning object with a single, focused learning outcome, the content to address the learning outcome, and formative assessment questions with considerable feedback on responses. The content and assessments have been tested, teaching with both undergraduate and postgraduate students.

How to use this book for students

Following each section are questions about concepts mentioned in the section. Answer the questions by writing down an answer and then consult the end of the text for suggested answers and more detailed responses.

Undergraduate science programmes, biological sciences, genetics, ecology, environmental sciences, psychological sciences

The text can be used as a formal guide for delivering lectures on the topics covered in each section. We have found setting the lecture in the style of a question can aid the discussion and identify key areas of focus that are of interest to the audience.

Medical, dental, nursing, midwifery programmes

The text can be used as a reference tool for delivering tutorials on the topics covered. We have found setting the discussion of topics in the style of a tutorial can aid the application of concepts to more immediate experiences of the medical student, either as experienced in the hospital setting or their previous personal experiences with illness.

Master's and doctoral level students, public health, primary care, researcher training, psychology and psychiatry

Each section stands alone and can be used as a single focus of discussion. The examples used to illustrate the concepts are designed to be generalizable to the master's students' own experience and interactions with patients. A greater focus on how to implement and integrate the ideas covered in each section with the master's students' experience should be a main focus here.

1 Foundations of Epidemiology

Sections in this chapter are aimed to provide a foundation for statistical epidemiology. The aim is to give an overview of the science and some of the history, and describe the important role epidemiology has to play. We hope this section will inspire students to pursue learning about statistical epidemiology through understanding its importance to society.

1.1 An Introduction

- Pre-requisite sections: None.
- Learning outcome: By the end of this section you should be able to define epidemiology and some important concepts used in the discipline.

In the academic tradition, let's start with a definition: Last described epidemiology as 'the study of the distribution and determinants of health-related states ...' (Last, 2000). This definition contains key ingredients of the discipline. One of these, 'health', is a commonly used term but you may not have considered what it means. In 1948, the World Health Organization described health as 'a complete state of physical, mental and social well-being, and not merely the absence of disease or infirmity' (WHO, 1948).

This definition has stood the test of time, with its subsequent adoption by public health and science. However, Last's definition used the term 'health-related states' which is more specific, and more properly leads us to ask 'what is a good measure of health?' These states, or measures of health, include occurrence of disease, death, the use of health services such as an admission to a hospital, health behaviours such as exercise, reaction to treatments such as an allergic reaction to penicillin, accidents and many more. Over the history of this discipline, specific terms have been developed to assist the exchange of ideas and findings. Some of the core definitions are given in Box 1.1.

Statistical epidemiology is an emerging branch of the discipline, integrating epidemiology and biostatistics to bring more statistical rigour to the field of epidemiology. The discipline recognizes the importance of applied statistics, especially with respect to the context in which statistical methods are appropriate or inappropriate. These concepts, such as the use of causal diagrams and bias, will be explored.

Measuring the distribution by time, place and person

Last's definition has two key activities in relation to the outcomes of interest: measuring the distribution and identifying the determinants. Before an epidemiologist can

Box 1.1. Commonly used terms in epidemiology

Aetiology: The study of the cause, or causes, of a disease.

Case: A person with a disease of interest.

Cause: See Exposure.

Disease: Not straightforward to define, but at its most generic disease is the impairment of normal physiological function. This is also referred to as an outcome or illness.

Exposure: A factor that a person experiences. Factors could include chemicals (e.g. cigarette smoke), biological entities (e.g. virus), physical entities (e.g. ultraviolet radiation), behavioural patterns (e.g. visiting the doctor), and/or a myriad of social and cultural customs.

Morbidity: Illness, loss of ability, disease.

Mortality: Loss of life, death.

Outcome: An event that a person experiences. This event interests the epidemiologist.

Risk factor: An exposure that may lead to an outcome.

---

make headway with identifying the determinants, or causes, of an outcome of interest, the first stop is to measure its distribution. This involves counting the people with the outcome, such as the number of people with a disease, or the number of deaths. Whilst knowledge of the volume of the outcome is important for managing resources, such as providing sufficient healthcare professionals to deal with an outbreak of a disease, it is only the start. We make progress by dividing these counts by the important characteristics of the people that we are surveying.

To do this an epidemiologist will often examine the distribution by time, by place and by person. This is the 'epidemiological triad'. As an example, let us consider a large number of cases of cancer, often referred to as a 'cluster', in the United States that has caused controversy (Steinberg *et al.*, 2007). The place where these cases were discovered is Fallon in Nevada, the time is 1997–2003, and the persons are children. Fifteen children were diagnosed with acute lymphoblastic leukaemia over these 7 years in Fallon. The key information from the triad is the place, as Fallon houses the naval aviation base made famous by the movie *Top Gun*, raising a political controversy on the safety and placement of the base.

Knowing the causes of an outcome influences society

When we think of things that determine an illness we are asking the question 'What is causing this disease?' In this sense we need to consider what range of exposures a person has had that may have helped bring this disease out now as opposed to at any other time. We are looking for the clues to the cause of disease, with the aim to reduce its mortality and morbidity. These clues have already led to interventions that are effective in improving health; we will go into more detail in Section 1.3.

Epidemiology can assist individuals, members of the public, you and me, make a myriad of decisions in their day, from whether to have a cigarette or have that cheeseburger for lunch. Epidemiologists also assist health professionals in completing the clinical picture, documenting the course of a disease from the beginning of an outbreak to the end. As we will see from the birth of modern epidemiology, the search for a cause can greatly influence public policy and business practices and change the course of something as basic as the provision of water.

Epidemiology can involve the urgent chasing of an unexpected occurrence of disease, where time is of the essence and a deployment to the field is required. This has happened many times; a recent example is the epidemic of severe acute respiratory syndrome (SARS) during 2002–2003 which required a concerted effort to measure the disease distribution, work out how to implement interventions, and follow the epidemic until it was under control. In contrast to the acute mobilization of resources, epidemiology can be a time-consuming trawl through mountains of data. We sift through the cloudy haze of anecdote and superstition to end up at a place where no other person has been. The depth of this haze is increasing; the main causes of death for the human population are due to chronic disease rather than the infectious nature of illness, which took the lives of so many of our ancestors. Chronic disease develops over an extended period, and is rarely due to a single factor.

Epidemiology has a long history

To examine the development of the science of epidemiology we start back in history with the ancient Egyptians. Imhotep was the chief magician of the court of Dozer, who reigned 2630–2611 BC, and must have been a physician of considerable skill whereby he attained demigod status 100 years after his death. He appears to have been the first physician and seems to have set the stage for this position having a great deal of power associated with it.

In China, Emperor Huang Ti (the Yellow Emperor) wrote the canon of internal medicine called the Nei Ching in the 3rd millennium BC. As the earliest surviving work on Chinese medicine it outlines the understanding of Chinese medicine including illness, medicines, diagnosis and treatment.

Hammurabi was a Babylonian king in the 18th century BC, who employed an extreme code which included laws relating to the practice of medicine. Penalties for failure were severe, for example, 'If the doctor, in opening an abscess, shall kill the patient, his hands shall be cut off'.

Until Hippocrates of Cos, who was born around the 4th century BC, became a physician in ancient Greece, medicine was indistinct from other fields that it had traditionally been associated with, notably theology and philosophy. He is one of the most outstanding figures in the history of medicine with some calling him the 'father of medicine' in recognition of his lasting contributions to the field. Hippocrates set the basis for the empirical sciences moving away from a requirement for spiritual faith. Through observation as a way to obtain knowledge about health, he looked to his environment highlighting the need for good sanitation, personal hygiene and diet, noting 'let food be thy medicine; and let thy medicine be food'. The concept of balance, as applied to personal health, also began at this time with the four fluids, blood, yellow bile, black bile, and phlegm, which needed to be in balance otherwise poor health would result.

Medicine was intertwined with astrology and other non-scientific superstitions in the middle ages. Manuscripts have been found that contain pen and ink drawings with explanatory texts. Including the earth and seven planets, they detail how each sign of the zodiac is related to a specific part of the body. Bloodletting charts, instructions on the best days to draw blood and the body points from which to draw it are also included. This contrasts starkly with the next section on the power of observations.

Observation powered advances in medical science

We now skip forward in history, to a French physician, Guillaume de Baillou (1538–1616), whose work in compiling a clear account of disease epidemics from 1570 to 1579 was the first of its kind since Hippocrates. He is credited with describing specific plagues, such as whooping cough in 1578, which is caused by *Bordetella pertussis* and involved an upper respiratory tract infection with a characteristic cough. Four years after his death, an Englishman named John Graunt (1620–1674) was born. He studied death records kept by London parishes, going back to 1532; he noted certain phenomena appeared regularly. In his *Natural and Political Observations Made upon the Bills of Mortality* (1672), Graunt aimed 'to know how many die before they can speak, or how many live past any assigned number of years' (p.29). He also classified death rates according to cause of death (Graunt, 1939). Among these, he included observations on overpopulation and sex: the urban death rate exceeded the rural, male birth rates were higher than for females, and the mortality rate was higher in males. He concluded that the population was divided almost evenly between the sexes. Predictions of the percentage of persons that were to live to each successive age and their life expectancy year by year was also calculated using what is known as the life table.

Thomas Sydenham (1624–1689), a British physician, also made significant contributions to clinical medicine and epidemiology. Emphasizing the same type of detailed observations on patients Hippocrates favoured, he was among the first to describe scarlet fever and St. Vitus' dance (also named Sydenham's chorea). In Italy, Bernardino Ramazzini (1633–1714) described outbreaks of chickpea poisoning (1690) and malaria (1690–1695). These observations show that advancements in medicine were gaining momentum. Edward Jenner (1749–1823) observed that a person who had suffered from cowpox, a harmless disease that could be contracted from cattle, could not contract smallpox. Smallpox was a major killer in its time, and Jenner with the assistance of a dairymaid, Sarah Nelmes with fresh cowpox lesions on her hand, was able to inoculate an 8-year-old boy, James Phipps who had never had smallpox, with cowpox. Although Phipps became slightly ill over the next days he did not develop smallpox. Jenner then inoculated the boy with smallpox matter, and no disease developed.

These descriptions show us the power of observation. We base the successful development of making a diagnosis and selecting a treatment, on someone with a keen eye for patterns. Observations are a first part of the scientific method (see Section 1.2). It has been said 'making observations is the first duty of the citizen' (Professor Sir Richard Friend, interview with Vega in 2005) and making observations is also one of the most important roles of an epidemiologist.

Tell it to the people

One of the major difficulties faced by epidemiologists in both modern and ancient times is the problem of telling people about their findings. The progression of science is generally a difficult battle where a new hypothesis, or set of observations, must supersede an existing idea. This inevitably leads to a conflict where people, personalities, business and politics are involved. Max Planck is paraphrased saying that 'science proceeds one funeral at a time', in other words that we progress once younger scientists qualify and older scientists retire or die.

An early practitioner of epidemiology, John Snow, known for his work on anaesthesia and for his work on the transmission of cholera, had a battle with the authorities to get his message heard. Snow was born in York in 1813 (Fig. 1.1) and after a conventional upbringing he became a physician in London. He calculated dosages for chloroform and gave this to Queen Victoria during two childbirths.

A large number of deaths from cholera in London prompted him to explore the spatial distribution of these deaths, and he discovered a preponderance of cases around contaminated water coming from the Broad Street pump in London. Our understanding now is that a bacterium causes cholera, and it is important to remember that the cause was then believed to be due to air pollution. The discovery that cholera was caused by contaminated water is a defining moment in epidemiology. However, Snow faced opposition, particularly from the water supply companies, but through speaking with local residents and the council Snow managed to persuade the council to disable the water pump by removing the handle.

Florence Nightingale (1820–1910) worked as a nurse in the Crimean war. She observed that more soldiers died in hospital after the battle than during any battle. She also noted improvements in sanitation were associated with improved outcomes. She used a modified pie chart, known as a polar diagram, and other ways to demonstrate her findings which contributed to Nightingale becoming the first female member of the Royal Statistical Society and later an honorary member of the American Statistical Association. She is credited with using applied statistics to bring about evidence-based change in health delivery and improvements in health.

A further pioneer in the area of investigation of the influence of the environment on disease was Alice Hamilton (1869–1970), an American pathologist, who became

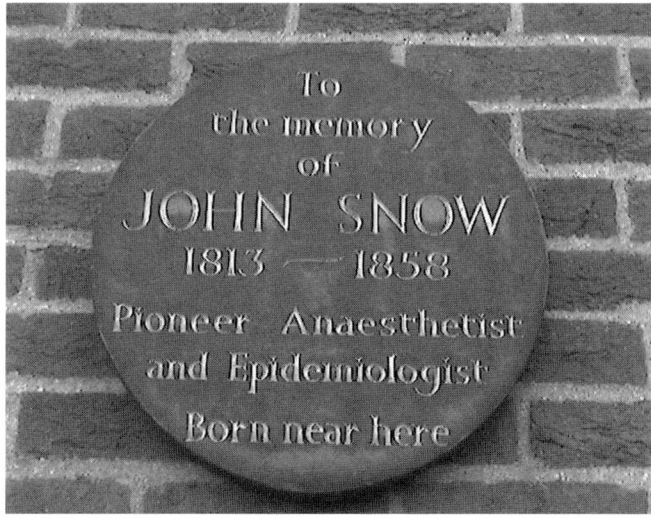

Fig. 1.1. Plaque commemorating the birthplace of John Snow.

known for her research on industrial diseases. She actively publicized the danger to workers' health from industrial toxic substances such as lead and mercury, contributing to the passage of workers' compensation laws and to the development of safer working conditions. Two individuals at this time made significant contributions to the study of yellow fever. Yellow fever can kill at an astounding rate if a person is not immunized. Max Theiler (1899–1972) was a South African-born microbiologist who developed a vaccine against yellow fever, for which he received the 1951 Nobel Prize for physiology or medicine.

In the modern day, Nathan Wolfe, an American virologist and epidemiologist, conducted studies on transmission of infectious viruses such as those closely related to human immunodeficiency virus (HIV). Wolfe also played a central role in establishing the Global Viral Forecasting Initiative (GVFI), a programme designed to monitor the transmission of viruses from animals to humans in countries worldwide.

There are sub-disciplines of epidemiology

There are many sub-disciplines of epidemiology, where specialisms have wished to take the methods of epidemiology and extend them to a specific area. Sometimes these are based in disease groups, such as cancer epidemiology. Others are based on special methods.

The term 'molecular epidemiology' was coined in 1973 (Kilbourne, 1973) to encompass the use of laboratory techniques to advance knowledge of the aetiology of disease. Molecular epidemiology can be used to examine exposure, diagnosis and processes of disease. Similarly 'genetic epidemiology' uses standard epidemiological techniques, along with some more specific to the sub-discipline, to explore the associations between genetics and disease. This includes identifying the common genetic variants in the population and the level of modification of risks to disease.

'Spatial epidemiology' uses the spatial methods from geography. John Snow was an early proponent of using maps to explore the putative risk factors for disease with successful results. Other sub-disciplines are interested in the exposures specifically rather than outcome, such as the epidemiology that examines the food intake of subjects, known as 'nutritional epidemiology'.

Summary

Epidemiology has a long history, but scientific discovery is not finished and the knowledge of diagnosis, disease process, causes, and treatment continues to grow. The epidemiologist's first job is to make observations, which has a long tradition in medicine. These observations may be related to the time, place and person, to inform the discovery of the determinants or cause of an outcome.

Self-test questions

Q 1.1.1: What makes up the epidemiological triad?

Q 1.1.2: Which of these are possible causes of a disease?
A Outcome
B Exposure
C Risk factor
D Cluster

Q 1.1.3: Epidemiology is the study of:
A Geriatric diseases
B Outbreak of disease in populations
C Elephants
D Skin conditions

Q 1.1.4: In 1850s London how do you stop the spread of cholera?
A Disable the water pump by removing the handle
B Drink gin
C Hold your breath
D Wait for a cure

Q 1.1.5: Florence Nightingale was the first female member of which Royal Society?

1.2   Science and Its Methods

● Pre-requisite sections: 1.1.
● Learning outcome: By the end of this section you should be able to define scientific method and its role in science and health research.

Many of us were taught 'science' at school. But do many of us stop to think what a science is? There are common misunderstandings of what science is, and what a scientist does (see Box 1.2). The aim of this section is to explore the way in which science is conducted and how knowledge is gained, using a process known as the scientific method. We will consider some examples of the scientific method and compare these to other methods people use to make decisions.

Box 1.2. Defining science

What defines science? Is it what scientists do? If so, how could you define a scientist? It can be hard to consider what clearly defines what science is that also reflects its breadth. How about defining science as physics, biology and chemistry? That leaves out social science and medical science. How about science being what is conducted in a laboratory? That omits studies like drug trials in the community. You could even say that science is the combined wealth of knowledge from human kind, but this includes historical information and knowledge of literature, neither of which are sciences.

To use an analogy to address the problem, how might we define chess? It is a game with pieces that move on a board. The pieces are moved on the basis of a series of rules. We can apply this to define science: it is a field of exploration defined by rules, which are laid down and collectively known as the scientific method. (But a word of warning, Einstein in 1953 said, 'Whoever undertakes to set himself up as a judge in the field of Truth and Knowledge is shipwrecked by the laughter of the gods.'!)

Science and epidemiological research in particular usually involves the cooperation of many people. The level of cooperation necessarily leads to difficulties in controlling all possible variation in the research. Unlike other forms of science, which have greater control over the environment around them, for example laboratory-based studies, epidemiologists are unable to control many of the variables they study. Other limitations include the need to maintain confidentiality for human participants in a study, ethical issues based on culture or belief, legal issues and claims for compensation, budgetary restraints, and access to participants.

A struggle for many academic disciplines is in the development of a common language, free from the jargon that divides and interferes with cooperation. By describing the scientific method, we will discover the words that are common amongst the sciences. Box 1.3 gives the definitions for many of these.

Scientific method underpins the way we do science

Scientific method is a process aimed at developing new knowledge and testing the usefulness of things which we presume to know. The method, depicted in Fig. 1.2, begins when a scientist makes an interesting observation. An observation is an activity where we record an event through using human senses or instruments. This may lead to a measurement of the magnitude or quantity of the entity under observation. A scientist must be aware that when you observe a process, the action of observation may affect the process you are observing. We call this the observer effect, and it may lead to a different measurement compared to the outcome of an unobserved process. A simple example is that it is not possible to measure the air pressure in a tyre without releasing some of that pressure.

Let us use a hypothetical situation to explore the scientific method. Fran, a budding scientist, sees a white rabbit for the first time, in a field. The first stage in the method is to propose what is known as a hypothesis. A hypothesis is a statement explaining what the scientist thinks is happening, based on the scientist's observation. Fran may propose the hypothesis that 'all rabbits are white'. This hypothesis fits with the observation she has made.

Box 1.3. Scientific definitions

Empirical method: the collection of data under natural, non-experimental conditions.

Hypothesis: an explanation of an observation.

Law: a statement that expresses a fundamental relation or rule.

Measurement: the acquisition of an estimate of the magnitude or quantity of the entity under observation.

Observation: an activity where an event is recorded through using human senses or instruments.

Operational definition: the operations or events that go into making an observation.

Reliability: extent to which a method gives consistent measurements.

Theory: a collection of observations, laws and concepts.

Validity: how closely a measurement corresponds with the true value.

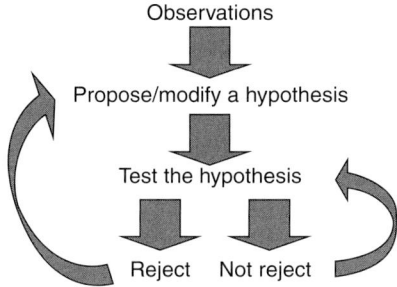

Fig. 1.2. Scientific method.

As Fran is a good scientist, she will then test her hypothesis. There are many ways to test a hypothesis. In our example, to test her hypothesis Fran travels to a neighbouring field where she observes another white rabbit. Using scientific method Fran is unable to reject the hypothesis that she first proposed: the new observation 'fits' with her original hypothesis. However, she does not finish here; in Fig. 1.2 an arrow returns to testing the hypothesis and so she must continue to test her hypothesis.

Let us assume that in a third field she now sees a brown rabbit. She must reject her first hypothesis and either propose a new hypothesis, or at least modify the existing one. She elects to modify the hypothesis to 'all rabbits are either white or brown'. Fran is not finished; she now continues to test her new hypothesis. As you can infer, the scientific method does not have a finishing point. We will discuss this unsatisfactory issue in Section 2.1.

A hypothesis is different to a scientific law or theory. A law is a statement of a fundamental relation or rule that expresses a scientific principle. The process of inductive reasoning confirms scientific laws. It is common to amend laws to fit more and more specific situations as science progresses. We are not aware of any laws in epidemiology. A scientific theory proposes a mechanism or explanation of phenomena, comprising a collection of concepts and laws. Epidemiology and science generally, confines itself to the hypothesis as this provides the precision required to advance our knowledge.

Hypotheses must be falsifiable

All hypotheses, and by extension science, must be 'falsifiable': you must be able to reject a hypothesis as not correct. A good definition of a falsifiable hypothesis is one where it is possible to take two positions on a statement, one true and one false. Nothing that cannot be falsified can be tested. If a researcher deems a statement not to be falsifiable, such as those used in belief systems, it does not mean it is not a useful statement, but it is not applicable to science.

The condition of falsifiability means that the scientist must be able to test a hypothesis and reject it if it is inconsistent with their observations. If there were observations that did not fit with the hypothesis then the hypothesis is false. (As Thomas Henry Huxley (1825–1895) said, 'Science is organized common sense where many a beautiful theory was killed by an ugly fact.'!) The degree of clarity and precision of a hypothesis has a bearing on whether it is falsifiable. It is easier to falsify a clear, precise and indeed an extreme hypothesis than one that is vague and not complete.

For the health sciences, falsifiability often leads to controversy. Previous medical advice based on an earlier hypothesis may be changed because the hypothesis was subsequently rejected and a new hypothesis has been proposed. It is understandably difficult for patients when the advice provided by medical practitioners changes. However, this is science succeeding by further clarifying a hypothesis. An example is the change in prescribing practice for hormone replacement therapy (HRT) around the time of the menopause, which was widely used to prevent osteoporosis. Subsequent scientific research shows that the risk for cancer, heart attack and stroke outweighs the benefits of the therapy (Boorstin and Waterman, 1995). Advice to general practitioners in the UK, and globally, changed to reflect this, by restricting HRT to a maximum of three years. This generated controversy at the time both in the media and for patients confused by a change in the advice.

A scientist starts with a null hypothesis

The first stage for testing a hypothesis is to define a 'null hypothesis' which proposes a position that is opposite to the relationship you are interested in. For example, when the hypothesis you wish to test proposes a relationship between two things, then the null hypothesis would propose no relationship. The null hypothesis for Fran, after her first observation, was that all rabbits were white.

The next stage is to propose the 'alternative hypothesis', which usually proposes a particular relationship between the two things we are interested in. It is important that the null and alternative hypotheses are defined in advance of testing them. The scientist then collects data that rejects the alternative hypothesis, hence confirming that the null hypothesis is true. So when Fran finds a brown rabbit, this makes the initial null hypothesis impossible, and therefore determines that the null hypothesis was false. If Fran had not found any rabbits except ones with white fur, then she would not have rejected the null hypothesis.

Hypotheses should be no more complex than required

A rule of thumb in scientific method is 'Occam's razor', named after a 13th century Franciscan friar William of Ockham, which is a concept that has been frequently stated by many thinkers throughout history. This principle states that a hypothesis should only be as complex as it needs to be to explain the observations. Fran demonstrates this with a simple initial hypothesis, that all rabbits are white. As happens frequently in science, further observations lead to the hypothesis becoming more complex, which is what happened to Fran. This still fits with Occam's razor.

Occam's razor is not a formalized part of scientific method. On the other hand, the principle of parsimony is a closely aligned statistical practice where we use the simplest model to explain data.

Science differs from everyday approaches

Hippocrates of Cos, discussed in Section 1.1, was the founder of the Hippocratic School of medicine. Credited with greatly advancing the systematic study of clinical medicine, Hippocrates summarized the extent of medical knowledge and prescribing by physicians through the Hippocratic Oath. His work contributed to translating medicine and health into a systematic domain, moving from subjective interpretations. These works set the basis for differentiating between everyday approaches and the study of medicine as a scientific discipline.

Marx provides some useful insights into the difference between the use of scientific method and the way people operate each day. The way people make sense of their world can be described as 'intuitive' (Marx, 1963). A person using the intuitive process learns and understands without the need for the approach to be broken down into a set of premises and these premises tested. Intuitive approaches can be quick and easy to use, however can be subject to the influence of illusion. Table 1.1 describes some of the differences between scientific and everyday approaches to situations.

A traditional approach to healing, in some cultures, is encapsulated by the saying 'the hair of the dog'. The ancient wisdom recommends placing hair from a rabid dog that bit you to cure the infection in the wound. This traditional approach, based on the concept of 'like cures like', is an erroneous approach to health. The consumption of alcohol when suffering from a hangover is an example with the aim to lessen the symptoms. This has a basis in intuition and experience as further alcohol does indeed alleviate some of the painful symptoms.

Other forms of intuition or subjective assessment are also incorrect. Fig. 1.3 shows two lines, where you can use an indirect measure involving using your eyes to guess the difference and make a comparison between the two lines. An empirical approach uses direct observations achieved by measuring the length. This is known as the Müller-Lyer illusion distortion and is caused when using your eyesight alone to measure (Müller-Lyer, 1886).

Table 1.1. Comparison of the aims of everyday and scientific approaches.

	Everyday approach	Scientific approach
General approach	Intuitive	Empirical
Observation	Casual, uncontrolled	Systematic controlled
Reporting	Biased, subjective	Unbiased, objective
Concepts	Ambiguous	Clear
Instruments	Inaccurate, imprecise	Accurate, precise
Measurement	Unknown validity or reliability	Valid and reliable
Hypothesis	Untestable	Testable
Attitude	Uncritical, accepting	Critical, unaccepting

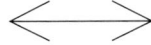

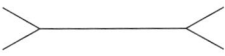

Fig. 1.3. Müller-Lyer illusion. Look at the images and choose which is longer.

Tricksters make good scientists

In many cultures, the trickster has played an important role in storytelling and myth. The trickster is a creature or god who behaves in a mischievous way, but accidentally or purposefully causes positive effects (Hyde, 1999). A well-known mythical trickster is Eshu, a deity from the Yoruba mythology, which forms the religious beliefs and practices of the Yoruba people of West Africa, chiefly Nigeria and Benin. Eshu is a god of chaos and trickery, a difficult teacher but a worthwhile guide.

Acting in a sceptical or questioning way is classically how a scientist should behave. Konrad Lorenz, an Austrian zoologist said 'It is a good morning exercise for a research scientist to discard a pet hypothesis every day before breakfast.' (Lorenz, 1966). This contains a trickster attitude, with an important message for the scientist: hypotheses are there to be thrown away, not to be held on to.

As Burt Rutan, the winner of the X-Prize, said: 'A true creative researcher has to have confidence in nonsense' (Rutan, 2004). This summarizes the trickster nature of science and scientists.

Observation and measurement are crucial to science

Empirical evidence comes from the collection of data, facts and observations. Empirical evidence based on observation under natural conditions should be contrasted with experimental evidence, which is based on manipulating the environment. The misconception that science is only done in a laboratory has some basis; a cornerstone of science is the effort that goes into clarity of observation. Scientists must be able to repeat the same observations allowing independent researchers to repeat the test of a hypothesis. For example, smoking is an exposure that epidemiologists often measure, but this is an imprecise concept. An epidemiologist decides whether they are looking at cigarette or pipe smoking, filtered or unfiltered cigarettes, the type of tobacco, manner (for example using a cigarette holder) and frequency of inhalation, and when and where the person smokes.

Measurements must be reliable and valid

Two aspects of measurements, validity and reliability, are often assessed side by side. The validity of a measurement refers to how closely a measurement corresponds to the truth. Reliability of a measurement is the extent to which a measurement gives consistent results. The term 'gold standard' refers to the best method available for producing a measurement we believe best or most close to the true value. Scientists must be careful using this term, as it is not possible to know the truth. However, scientists use logical arguments to justify a method as the gold standard.

Reliability involves freedom from random and systematic errors and furthermore the errors do not cause the measurement to lie systematically further from the truth. A test cannot have high validity unless it also has high reliability. Assessing reliability is often straightforward, through replication of a method. It is more difficult to assess validity, as we usually do not know the true value of a measure. It is possible to assess validity in some domains. For example, we assess the validity of a screening test for subsequent disease after sufficient time has elapsed for a disease to present.

Science needs statistics

Following the successful conduct of an epidemiology study, the scientist must use statistical analyses to make appropriate inference. Statistics and tests of statistical significance look to determine whether an event could have occurred by chance or randomly. In epidemiology, this may be when an exposure is not related to the development of a disease. We use statistical analyses to estimate the effects of the variables, and to assess levels of bias. Bias can be a particularly difficult issue to deal with and statisticians have developed some ingenious methods to ameliorate its effects.

From statistical analysis, we can start to make decisions about the options and indeed their utility. The statistics provide a background for policy makers to make decisions, for doctors to determine treatment options, to inform patients of the course of disease, and for the public to decide on risk.

Experiences of bad science

From time-to-time, mavericks appear in science, tricksters if you will. Some mavericks are shown to be correct, and others not. A fine line exists between a bad scientist and one who is questioning the establishment. A notorious case of bad science was in the controversy surrounding the vaccination of children against measles, mumps and rubella using a triple vaccine (MMR). Andrew Wakefield, a former surgeon in the United Kingdom, and colleagues published an article in *The Lancet* (Wakefield *et al.*, 1998) that proposed a new syndrome linking bowel disease, autism and the MMR vaccine. The entire study was based on 12 children, consisted of poor study design, and made claims beyond the scope of the study. This led to a loss in public confidence in the triple vaccine, and a dramatic loss of herd immunity; there have been small outbreaks and epidemics of these diseases. In 2010, Wakefield was removed from the UK register of doctors and his research has been discredited, meanwhile herd immunity is gradually recovering after a concerted effort by public health and government officials.

Gross (see Box 1.4) offers words of warning for science. Science is not a perfect solution to the questions that cause society problems. It is a process, a set of methods, by which an individual may find answers to difficult questions. Bad science can have

---

Box 1.4. Gross on science (Gross and Levitt, 1998, p. 45)

'Science is a highly elaborated set of conventions brought forth by one particular culture (our own) in the circumstances of one particular historical period; thus it is not, as the standard view would have it, a body of knowledge and testable conjecture concerning the 'real' world. It is a discourse, devised by and for one specialized 'interpretive community', under terms created by the complex net of social circumstance, political opinion, economic incentive and ideological climate that constitutes the ineluctable human environment of the scientist. Thus, orthodox science is but one discursive community among the many that now exist and that have existed historically. Consequently its truth claims are irreducibly self referential, in that they can be upheld only by appeal to the standards that define the 'scientific community' and distinguish it from other social formations.'

---

a dramatic effect on society, in the same way that good scientists can. Science retains, in the western world, a privileged position to advise the public and policy makers alike. This freedom needs to be weighed against the fairly rare cases of people wishing to further their own ambitions, for fame and money that can cause damage to society and to the reputation of science.

Summary

There is a formalized approach to making decisions using scientific method. Facts are acquired through observation and measurement, followed by a process of inductive reasoning to allow a hypothesis to be proposed. Then through a process of deduction, a scientist makes predictions.

The scientific method provides the test of what we consider true. In the absence of any real test it is easy to think you are progressing, following the well intentioned but fundamentally artificial guidelines of life and actually not progress. A false confidence develops. When a researcher presents the test, the illusion of competence is shattered, and people react, badly sometimes. It is all too easy to feel betrayed, let down and to 'blame the messenger'.

Self-test questions

Q 1.2.1: A scientist discovers that smoking cannabis may induce premature dementia. She then conducts a second study that was unable to reject her initial hypothesis. Following good scientific method should she:
A Conduct a third study to test the hypothesis
B Declare that her hypothesis is correct
C Reject her initial hypothesis and amend it

Q 1.2.2: An epidemiology study found that surfing in the sea was associated with gastrointestinal infection. Should a scientist:
A Accept this as true
B Test this again

Q 1.2.3: What is the null hypothesis?

Q 1.2.4: How do you define validity?

1.3   The Importance of Epidemiology

- Pre-requisite sections: 1.1.
- Learning outcome: By the end of this section you should move away from 'Epidemiology and public health has no relevance to me' towards 'I understand the importance of evidence-based scientific research of disease. I can see how it will have relevance to me as a clinician or scientist'.

Do you know why we spend money on epidemiology? Why charities and governments pay for epidemiology? What has it done for society? Does epidemiology have any impact on you, either personally or in your job? You may be asking these questions. To get you thinking about this, let's start with a simple question, which forms the core of this section.

Take a moment to think about this statement: 'Epidemiology has no impact on me.' Do you agree, disagree or are you undecided?

Imagine a world without epidemiology

Speaking with many different people, in different professions, suggests to us that it is difficult to convince the public of the relevance that the scientific study of populations and disease will have to you, to the public, or to patients. To illustrate the importance of epidemiology it is easier if you use your imagination to think of a world where epidemiology did not exist (Box 1.5).

We all benefit from public health and we need the science it is based on, including epidemiology: the study of where disease occurs, and why. The term is based on the ancient Greek 'epi demos logos', literally, 'the study upon the people'. It can be anything from finding out why there is an outbreak of a new disease – like a pandemic flu – to working out what things cause the diseases that kill the most people in a country. Public perception of such health research is important: support both financially and in individuals' involvement is crucial for its success.

Medicine as we know it would also be vastly different in a world with no epidemiology. There would be little understanding of disease; plagues of infection would rampage through the world because germ theory of disease would not have been proposed and tested; our water supply would still be contaminated causing outbreaks

---

Box 1.5. A world without epidemiology

Imagine a world that is identical to the one we live in in every way, except one. This world does not have epidemiology; it doesn't have epidemiologists.

What would this world be like? There may be some benefits: by spending no money on health research, this world would save significant funds. There would be no health warnings about smoking and no restrictions on where people could smoke – in this world Sir Richard Doll would not have worked on tobacco. There would also be no warnings about sunbathing and sunlamps and you would have free reign to drink as much alcohol and eat as much fat and salt as you liked, with no pressure to eat healthily. In this world there would be no epidemiologists telling the government how to prevent disease. Because there is no epidemiology, you wouldn't even know these activities are unhealthy. The downside emerges: as a result there would be much higher numbers of deaths from heart attacks from the fat and salt intake. Lung cancers would be epidemic from the smoking, liver disease would result from unlimited alcohol consumption and malignant melanoma would be more common due to no precautions in sunlight exposure. You would be spending far more money on trying to cope with the burden of disease rather than the cheaper route of prevention.

Support and funding for epidemiological research helps to reduce public health spending further along in time, but more importantly, prevents much human suffering.

of many diseases; smallpox would reign because vaccinations and other public health measures would not have been evaluated. People might still be wondering about the mysteries of illness and disease because they would not have the capacity to test and research any theories of cause and effect.

All of these discoveries, which we now take for granted, were made by scientists employing epidemiological research techniques. This world has been dramatically transformed by discoveries made by epidemiology. However, individuals tend to forget the huge advances made by scientific research, and epidemiology in particular.

Healthcare professionals need epidemiology

A scientist should understand the role that epidemiology plays in developing public policy, and interventions that are required to prevent disease. Epidemiology provides an evidence base with which to determine policy, however, of course as with all policy decisions there are many other competing aspects to the decision-making process. Clinicians have their role doctors play in both preventing and curing disease. William Mayo (1861–1939), a leader in medicine and one of the founders of the Mayo Clinic in the United States of America, is quoted as stating '... the aim of medicine is to prevent disease and prolong life, the ideal of medicine is to eliminate the need of a physician'.

The development of doctors' abilities and skills, both curative and preventative, has been a slow process. The historian Professor David Wootton describes how, until epidemiology and biostatistics progressed sufficiently in the twentieth century, doctors caused their patients more harm than good (Wootton, 2006). The medical profession has often been reluctant to investigate and implement potentially beneficial interventions for either treatment or prevention. A well-known example is the investigation of scurvy on naval ships during the 18th and 19th centuries. James Lind, a Scottish clinician, conducted a controlled trial of 12 sailors, split into six pairs; the pair who were given citrus fruit made a rapid recovery. He published these results in 1753 in *A Treatise of the Scurvy*. However, it was a further 40 years before ships' surgeons trialled the use of lemon juice to cure and prevent scurvy.

Why did this take so long? One reason for these delays was that clinicians did not trust in the abilities of the tools of epidemiology and biostatistics to inform clinical decisions. This has changed: medical, dental and nursing students are taught the importance of evidence based on epidemiological research throughout their medical training.

The development of evidence-based practice

Evidence-based practice (EBP), sometimes referred to as evidence-based medicine (EBM), aims to apply evidence from scientific research to diagnosis and treatment decisions. This approach is used in a wide range of clinical settings, including medicine, surgery, dentistry, nursing and psychology. It assesses the strength of the evidence, weighing the risks and benefits for proposed therapies and diagnostic testing. EBP also recognizes that individual factors, such as judgements about the quality of life must also be incorporated into the decision-making process for a practitioner.

The evidence used by EBP is systematically collected, statistical methods are applied to the evidence collected, and then experts in the field are employed to decide on the best approaches. This leads to meta-analysis and evidence-based guidelines. These may become organizational policy, such as shown in the development of treatment policies in the England and Wales using the National Institute of Health and Clinical Evidence (NICE) guidelines. Much of the scientific evidence that is collected, appraised and implemented comes from epidemiology.

Leaders in epidemiology

Hippocrates, introduced in Section 1.2 along with being considered an early founder of Western medicine, may also be considered a father of epidemiology. During ancient times people did not realize that a disease might be caused by an external influence. He published a treatise *On Airs, Waters, and Places* which considered environmental risk factors for disease (see Box 1.6). Hippocrates is credited with saying 'To know the causes of a disease and to understand the use of the various methods by which the disease may be prevented amounts to the same thing as being able to cure the disease.' Sometimes this can be difficult for clinicians, but it is essentially the same as the adage 'Prevention is better than cure'.

John Snow is considered by many to be the father of modern epidemiology, with his implementation of prevention strategies based on germ theory. This happened during the 19th century and he was an important pioneer in advancing germ theory and using the epidemiological toolkit to elucidate the cause of cholera.

One of the leading pioneers in twentieth century epidemiology was Professor Sir Richard Doll (1912–2005). In the 1940s cancer was considered by many to be a normal feature of the ageing process. During the post-war period there was a great deal of road building and the UK Medical Research Council was concerned that

---

Box 1.6. *On Airs, Waters, and Places* **by Hippocrates, written 400 BCE, translated by Francis Adams**

'On Airs, Waters, Places, that … whoever wishes to investigate medicine properly should proceed thus: in the first place to consider the seasons of the year, and what affects each of them produces. Then the winds, the hot and the cold, especially such as are common to all countries and then such as are peculiar to each locality. In the same manner, when one comes into a city to which he is a stranger, he should consider its situation, how it lies as to the winds and the rising of the sun; for its influence is not the same whether it lies to the north or the south, to the rising or to the setting sun.

One should consider most attentively the waters which the inhabitants use, whether they be marshy and soft, or hard and running from elevated and rocky situations, and then if satisfy and unfit for cooking: and the ground, whether it be naked and deficient in water, or wooded and well watered, and whether it lies in a hollow, confined situation, or is elevated and cold; and the made in which the inhabitants live, and what are their pursuits, whether they are fond of drinking and eating to excess, and given to indolence, or fond of exercise and labour.'

---

poisonous fumes from the tarmacadam used to rebuild roads damaged during the war might be causing cancer. Doll organized social workers to interview 649 men with suspected cancer of the lung, bowel or liver in hospital wards in London. Of these men, just two of the lung cancer patients were non-smokers, whilst hardly any of those with other diseases were smokers. This was a startling result, which was totally unexpected.

Rapidly publishing these results, in 1950 in the British Medical Journal, the conclusion was that 'smoking is a factor, and an important factor, in the production of carcinoma of the lung' (Doll and Hill, 1950). Doll and his co-author Hill were not content to stop here. Referring back to the description of scientific method (Section 1.2) they decided to try to refute their hypothesis with an improved research study. They set up a cohort study (see Section 3.7) to examine more closely the possible association between smoking and lung cancer, known as the British Doctors' cohort, in which 34,000 male doctors were questioned about their smoking habits. None of them had been diagnosed with lung cancer at the start of the study. This group was an excellent cohort to study as they were easy to trace, provided a good response rate and it was thought they were fairly honest about their smoking habits. They were also an affluent group that had a high level of smokers. The cohort of doctors was then followed to find out how long they lived for and the cause of their deaths.

The results from the British Doctors' cohort were published in 1954 and the results confirmed the link between smoking and lung cancer risk (Doll and Hill, 1954). The UK government called a news conference, and the then health minister Iain Macleod said 'It must be regarded as established that there is a relationship between smoking and cancer of the lung.' It is interesting to note that throughout the press conference the minister and most of the journalists were chain-smoking. The British Doctors' cohort has been followed for 50 years, and the final publication in 2004 showed that there was a 10 years loss in life expectancy between smokers and non-smokers.

Doll's legacy is undoubted. In the 50 years since the British Doctors' cohort study was published smoking has become considerably less popular. The majority of British adults smoked in 1954, whilst in 2004 this had dropped to 26%. Conservative estimates for England alone are that 6 million people have avoided premature death by not smoking. And this must count in the tens of millions worldwide.

Summary

Describing the importance of epidemiology to the health of society is not a straightforward task. One way is to consider a world without the discoveries made by epidemiology. Rates of mortality and morbidity would be much higher than they are now. The epidemiology conducted by Sir Richard Doll has had huge global impact, and many of us have a great deal to thank him for.

This is summed up by the motto for the John Hopkins Bloomberg School of Public Health: 'Protecting health, saving lives – millions at a time'. Now think back to the question at the start of this section: 'Epidemiology has no impact on me'. Has your attitude changed?

Self-test questions

Q 1.3.1: Richard Doll and Austin Bradford Hill designed the:
A British Dentists' cohort
B British Doctors' cohort
C British Nurses' cohort
D British Veterinary cohort

Q 1.3.2: How many people have avoided premature death by not smoking since the Doll study?
A 6
B 600
C 600,000
D 6,000,000

Q 1.3.3: What is the aim of evidence-based medicine?

Q 1.3.4: Which of the following things prevent scurvy?
A Lemon juice
B Rum
C Sea water
D A sea shanty

1.4   Samples and Populations

- Pre-requisite sections: 1.1, 1.3.
- Learning outcome: By the end of the section you should be able to define populations, the sampling process and assess the validity of inferences that can be made from samples.

A population is every member of a group of interest. For example, every person in the United Kingdom (UK) defines a population when we are interested in the UK. Human disease research is unusual in that most other forms of scientific research do not have the opportunity to examine a population. Imagine ecology research when a researcher wants to measure the migration of a population of ants; it is an almost impossible task to count all of the ants in a population.

Surveys, such as a national census, measure and count almost everyone in the human population at a particular point in time within a locality. The precise number of the population can be affected by daily migration in and out of an area, residential migration, and the fact some people will be difficult to trace. This is a complex set of factors influencing the definition of boundaries for a population.

A population is referred to as the denominator

In epidemiology the total population or the underlying people who we are interested in measuring, is often referred to as the denominator. This term is the same as used for the lower part of a fraction; the numerator is the top part. Large-scale population surveys of the denominator, such as a national census, are expensive to conduct, complicated to administer and, for these reasons, usually conducted by governments. The involvement of large organizations, with a wide range of competing interests in the questions asked, often leads to population surveys having limited utility for epidemiology.

Health research progresses at a pace that often means the large surveys will not be able to meet the deadline required. For example, one of the roles of an epidemiologist is to measure and record outbreaks of emerging diseases. An outbreak occurs over a short time scale, days, weeks or months, and the research needs to be rapidly completed; large-scale surveys are not able to respond quickly enough. Large-scale surveys also may miss some difficult-to-find parts of the population. These partly accessible groups may include homeless people and wealthy people not registered with a local health practitioner.

Progress is made through sampling a population

The challenges in surveying an entire population pragmatically lead a scientist to study a smaller subset: the sample. The sample is composed of 'sampling units', selected to gain a picture that is representative of the entire population. When the sample is representative of the population, it is possible to 'infer' properties of the population from properties of the sample. Inference is a fundamental aspect of science and determines the need for statistical analysis. The term 'population parameter' is used to define a property of the population estimated using a sample. The value calculated from the sample is the 'sample statistic'.

Illustrating the importance of sampling in medicine, imagine that the Director of Public Health for the city of Newcastle wished to ascertain the prevalence of smoking amongst adults in Newcastle. This, at first sight, seems a straightforward exercise. The population is all adults in Newcastle, a hard to define group of people. Defining and delimiting a population can stray into a philosophical discussion; where do you draw the boundary? Do you include all members of a population now or at an earlier time? Alternatively, should you define the population to include all members across history, or into the future? We will not pursue these discussions, but a scientist should at least be aware of them.

Returning to the Director of Public Health, a questionnaire could be sent to every household in the area, but the cost would be prohibitive. The Director knows that there is no need to do this and so samples from the population by sending a questionnaire to a random sample of addresses in Newcastle asking residents whether they smoke. The Director decided that she had enough money for 1000 postal questionnaires and let us imagine that of these 372 were returned: these form the sample. From the questionnaire, 148 people declared that they smoked tobacco. The prevalence of smoking in the sample is calculated as the number of smokers, 148, divided by the number of people the returns related to, 372. You can infer from this calculation that the prevalence in the population is 39.8%.

'Chance' results make samples prone to error

Differences between the sample and the population exist because of the selection of particular sampling units. For example, if you selected ten people on the street it is feasible that you could find they were all over 1.8 m in height. You would suspect this was due to sampling; it is unlikely that the population are all over 1.8 m in height. This is sampling error and we should be aware of the potential for bias in our inference. Extending this simple thought experiment, you should be able to see that if you sample 100 people, compared to the earlier sample of just ten, it is far less likely that your whole sample will contain only people over 1.8 m in height. This offers the insight that the larger the sample, the closer to the population as a whole the measurements will become.

Sampling methods are designed to minimize errors

The principles underlying sampling are similar to the principles of the scientific method. We aim to use a methodology that is systematic, objective and defined beforehand. Our sampling units must be in themselves independent from one another, unchanging over time and not removable once they are included in the sample. The unchanging quality is important, going to the heart of the scientific method, as it is systematic and defined so that other scientists using the same method are able to reproduce your results.

Our main aim is to use a system that avoids error and bias. How do we do this? Why are we sampling is perhaps the most important of the initial questions. We take a sample from a population when we are unable to take measurements from the entire population. We are assuming the difference between the sample and the entire population is not large. What advantages does this bring? Advantages of sampling are that it takes less time and labour and is less costly than measuring all the sampling units in a population.

How we design the sampling method will determine some of the aspects of error and bias. There are many different ways to categorize the methods used for obtaining a sample. One of the fundamental ways to differentiate them is by the influence of probability (see Box 1.7).

Non-random methods may not be representative

Methods that do not use randomization are useful for descriptive analysis and may be used in the early stages of research. They do not claim to produce samples that are

---

Box 1.7. Random numbers

Many scientific disciplines use random numbers to define probability, epidemiology is no different: random numbers are used to select sampling units. Epidemiologists need a way to generate the random numbers. Simple physical methods have been around for millennia, such as flipping a coin or picking coloured balls from a bag. Tables of random numbers have been published since the 1930s.

With the advent of modern computers, there was an opportunity to develop programs that could produce random selections between any numbers. These random number generators are based on algorithms, and therefore are known as pseudo-random. In other words, it is possible, knowing the start point, to actually calculate the next numbers making them predictable. As technology has progressed the Internet has allowed a return to using a random number that exists somewhere remote; the scientist can use these numbers transmitted.

---

representative of the population but can provide rich data. If an epidemiologist were to try to use a non-random sample to infer properties of the population, then a deep understanding of the topic must be used and always with caution. The non-random methods are generally a less expensive way to sample, owing to the natural systems in place that allow us to easily select and recruit the sample. Non-random sampling techniques include:

1. Purposive, purposeful or judgemental sampling. As the name suggests there is a reason or purpose as to why we select sampling units. We choose units rich in information for in-depth study. Several types of purposive sampling techniques have been developed and identified. For example, a scientist may choose a sample with deviant or heterogeneous properties, where the highly unusual characteristics of the sample may lead to insights. Alternatively, we choose a sample to give the most variation in the study characteristics.

2. Accidental or haphazard sampling. Easily accessible members of the sample are chosen which gives a form of purposeful sampling that adds an element of randomness and therefore reduces the opportunity for bias.

3. Snowball sampling. The researcher identifies a unit of interest. For example, you may select a person and then ask them to recommend another person, such as a friend. This is a method used extensively in market research for commercial products, and does allow the recruitment of rich sampling units.

Random methods aim to be representative

Random methods of sampling at their simplest ensure that each unit has an equal probability of selection. This method, compared to non-random methods, is accurate, reliable and representative. Random methods also provide answers that are more generalizable. The downside is the extra time and resources required to identify the sampling frame and to recruit from it.

1. Simple probability sampling. All units have an equal chance of being selected using simple methods, such as randomly drawing numbered balls from a bag (the 'lottery method'), to using random number generation by a computer (see Box 1.7). Obtaining simple random sample units involves choosing units in such a way that each unit in the population has an equal chance of selection. A simple random sample is free from sampling bias. If a person untrained in statistics is collecting the sample, then instructions may be misinterpreted and selections poorly made. Using a random number generator to select a sampling unit from a list, assign each unit a random number (often between 0 and 1) and select the unit with the lowest number.

2. Systematic probability sampling. Instead of using a list of random numbers, data collection is simpler by selecting a unit after discarding a fixed number of other units after the first unit is chosen randomly. Care must be taken as there may be underlying systematic structure to the lists of sampling units. Other types include multi-stage sampling, multi-phase, area sampling, spatial and longitudinal sampling. For example, there are 100 students in your class. You want a sample of 20 from these 100 and you have their names listed on a piece of paper in alphabetical order. If you choose to use systematic random sampling, divide 100 by 20, you will get 5. Randomly select any number between 1 and 5. Suppose the number you have picked

is 4, that will be your starting number. You then select student number 4. From there you will select every 5th name until you end up with 20 selected students.

3. Stratified random sampling. Using stratified random sampling the population you are interested in is divided into groups, known as strata, and a unit that makes up the sample is drawn from each stratum. Strata occur naturally like the sex of a person, or are created artificially such as defining a family as people who share a house. A proportionate sample uses a population divided into strata and a random sample is taken from each stratum. As the name suggests a disproportionate sample takes more units from a stratum for a particular purpose. Both forms of stratified random sampling are useful when you require sampling units from all groups or strata. Other advantages are that it is an economical and straightforward way to provide a sample with high representativeness that you may not necessarily get from simple random sampling.

For example, a population may be divided into educational strata for sampling. A person with 10 years of education will be in group A, between 10 and 20 group B and between 20 and 30 group C, all referred to as strata. You can then randomly select from each stratum a given number of units which may be based on proportion. Let's assume group A has 100 persons while group B has 50, and C has 30. You may decide you will take 10% of each. So you end up with ten from group A, five from group B and three from group C.

4. Cluster sampling. The population is divided into 'clusters', groups which contain all elements of the broader population, and a sample of the groups is selected. Data is collected from the units within each selected cluster. This can be done for every sampling unit in each selected cluster or a sub-sample of sampling units may be selected within each of these clusters.

For example, a sample could be taken from final year high school students measuring their knowledge of human papillomavirus (HPV) and cervical cancer. A cluster may be a village, or a school or a state. So you decide all the elementary schools in New York State are clusters. You want 20 schools selected. You can use simple or systematic random sampling to select the schools, and then every school selected becomes a cluster. You may then interview all students or randomly select students on their knowledge of HPV.

When do we stop?

Knowing when to stop recruiting people into your study is an important aspect of research (see Box 1.8). There is no perfect way to determine how large your sample should be. Before starting a study the scientists determine the necessary sample size. Completing power analysis before a study commences can reduce time and resources carrying out a study which has only a small chance of finding a significant effect. From a sampling perspective, we do not waste time and resources testing more subjects than are necessary to detect an effect.

Different designs of epidemiology studies have different equations and methods for calculating the required size of a sample. Qualitative research presents difficult decisions of choosing a sample size. Unlike quantitative research, there are no definite rules to be followed, depending on what you want to know. With fixed resources, which are always the case, you can choose to study one specific phenomenon in depth with a smaller sample size, or a bigger sample size when seeking wide breadth in the information collected. In purposeful sampling, the sample should be judged on the basis of the purpose and rationale for each study and the sampling strategy used to achieve the study's purpose. The validity, meaningfulness and insights generated from qualitative inquiry have more to do with the information richness of the cases selected and the observational/analytical capabilities of the researcher than with sample size.

In an unconstrained world sample size depends on the nature of the analysis to be performed, the desired precision of the estimates one wishes to achieve, the kind and number of comparisons that will be made, the number of variables that have to be examined simultaneously and how heterogeneous a population is sampled. For example, if the key analysis of a randomized experiment consists of computing averages for experimental participants in a project and comparing differences, then a small sample may be adequate. In contrast, for observational research relevant variables have to be controlled statistically because groups differ by factors other than chance. This often leads to larger sample size being required.

More technical considerations suggest that the required sample size is a function of the precision of the estimates one wishes to achieve, the variability one expects to find in the population and the statistical level of confidence one wishes to use.

Summary

A sample is intended to be an unbiased and representative measure of a population and is taken when we are unable to study the entire population. The sample may be selected using simple random numbers, or more complex methods such as cluster randomized sampling may be employed. The size of the sample determines the level of sampling error in the data.

The size of the sample determines the level of sampling error in the data. Defining sample size is an important part of an epidemiology study, and this should be done preferably before the start of the study.

Self-test questions

Q 1.4.1: Why does an epidemiologist need to create a sample?

Q 1.4.2: What are the disadvantages of measuring the whole population?

Q 1.4.3: Which of these are random methods of sampling?
A Purposive sampling
B Snowball
C Cluster

1.5   Observational and Experimental Studies

- Pre-requisite sections: 1.1.
- Learning outcome: By the end of this section you should be able to describe the differences between observational and experimental research.

Albert Einstein said that the 'Development of Western Science is based on two great achievements: the invention of the formal logical system by the Greek philosophers, and the discovery of the possibility to find out causal relationships by systematic experiment.' (quoted in Boorstin and Waterman (1995)).

There is an important distinction between studies that make observations and studies that conduct experiments. It is possible for researchers to use both types of study to examine many research questions. The reason that one or other is used is most often due to feasibility: this will become clearer later in this section as we discuss economic, ethical and cultural issues and their relationship with research.

The experiment is one method to pursue science

Within the scientific method framework, an experiment is a method for investigating causal relationships among variables. You can derive the word experiment from the Latin 'experiri' meaning to 'to try out'. It allows us to collect data to help solve practical problems and to demonstrate that a hypothesis is not correct. A 'controlled experiment' generally compares the results obtained from an experimental sample against a control sample. We intend the control sample to be identical to the experimental sample except for the one aspect whose effect is under test, the 'independent variable'. A good example would be a drug trial. The people receiving the drug would be the experimental sample; the ones not receiving the trial drug would form the control sample.

Once we form two, or more, equivalent groups, the scientist treats them identically except for the one variable that he or she wishes to isolate. The goal of the experiment is to measure the response to a given stimulus by a test method. It is important that one knows all factors in an experiment. It is also important that the results are as accurate as possible. If we carefully conduct an experiment, the results either disprove or do not disprove the hypothesis under test. An experiment can never 'prove' a hypothesis, it can only disprove or not, and when it does not it adds support to the hypothesis. One repeatable experiment that provides a counterexample can disprove a hypothesis.

When you conduct an experiment, it is good practice to have several replicate samples for the test you are performing. 'Replication' of the results is an essential aspect of experiments as it ensures that other scientists can recreate the experiment – checking that the experimental method works and that the results are similar. It also provides the evidence that the experiment was not a 'one-off', that the results were not a unique or aberrant event. To be able to replicate an experiment protects science from fraud. To be generally accepted, experiments must be repeatable by others.

Laboratory-based experimental science often attempts to have both a 'positive control' and a 'negative control'. A negative control is one where the scientist is certain that the experiment will fail. We contrast this with a positive result where the scientist is certain the experiment will succeed. In epidemiology, these are not straightforward to design. The positive control assures the scientist that the experiment is able to produce a positive result. This may be important, especially when none of the experimental samples produce a positive result.

Natural experiments use naturally occurring circumstances

The term experiment usually implies a controlled experiment designed by a researcher and often taking place in a laboratory. Sometimes controlled experiments are prohibitively difficult or impossible. For example, some forms of intervention are not ethical, such as testing mobile phone use and brain tumours in children. In this case, researchers may resort to 'natural experiments', also called 'quasi-experiments'. The word 'quasi' means 'as if' or 'almost', so a quasi-experiment means almost a true experiment. Natural experiments rely solely on observations of the variables of the system under study, rather than manipulation of just one or a few variables as occurs in controlled experiments.

An example of a natural experiment occurred in Helena, Montana from June 2002 to December 2002 when a smoking ban was brought into effect in public places. The rate of heart attacks dropped by 60% while the smoking ban was in effect (Sargent *et al.*, 2004). The experiment could not disprove the hypothesis that smoking has no effect on the rate of heart attacks. This would not be ethical or financially viable to be done as a fully designed experiment.

To the degree possible, a natural experiment generates data about a system in such a way that contribution from all variables can be determined. The effects of variation in other important variables remain approximately constant.

Thought experiments may be used to replace physical experiments

'Thought experiments' employ imaginary situations to help us understand the way things really are. Understanding comes through reflection upon this imaginary situation. We do not use thought experiments extensively in epidemiology. They are more common in physics, where some questions are extremely difficult to explore using standard experimentation. Thought experimentation is not an empirical process: experiments are conducted within the imagination, and never in fact. In physics and other sciences, some famous thought experiments date from the 19th and 20th centuries, but examples can be found at least as early as Galileo.

Galileo is supposed to have conducted an experiment to demonstrate objects fall at the same rate regardless of their mass. This key experiment in the history of modern science challenged the view of Aristotle. This is widely thought to have been a straightforward physical demonstration, involving climbing up the Leaning Tower of Pisa and dropping two heavy weights off it, whereas it was also a logical demonstration, using the 'thought experiment' technique (see Box 1.9).

Scientists may use a thought experiment prior to a real experiment in the physical world. One hope is that the thought experiment will clearly offer results that will make conducting the physical experiment unnecessary. Scientists also use thought experiments when particular physical experiments are impossible to conduct, such as Einstein's thought experiment of chasing a light beam, leading to Special Relativity. This is a unique use of a scientific thought experiment, in that it was never carried out, but led to a successful theory, proven by other empirical means.

Einstein's influence went further than this, introducing new ways of doing 'thought experiments' mainly for theoretical science. Einstein has changed the way we think about science: he inspired a whole generation of scientists to change the way they thought about experiments, not requiring new more complex experiments (Norton, 2005). More than this, he questioned the certainty with which scientists viewed what they 'knew' about the world, showing them that things were not necessarily what they seemed.

In Box 1.5 we used a thought experiment to demonstrate the importance of epidemiology to the public. It is often not possible to explain the importance of epidemiology, because the general public forget rapidly how things were before the scientific discoveries made by epidemiologists. This was a thought experiment, which did not require any manipulation of the real world, as the conclusions are drawn through reasoned thought.

Box 1.9. Galileo's dialogue on gravity

The following is from Galileo's *Discorsi e dimostrazioni matematiche, intorno à due nuove scienze (Two New Sciences)* (Galileo, 1638), and takes the form of a dialogue between Salviati, who represents Galileo's views, and Simplicio, who argues against him. It is an example of the power of the thought experiment in demonstrating a mathematical argument.

Salviati: If then we take two bodies whose natural speeds are different, it is clear that on uniting the two, the more rapid one will be partly retarded by the slower, and the slower will be somewhat hastened by the swifter. Do you not agree with me in this opinion?

Simplicio: You are unquestionably right.

Salviati: But if this is true, and if a large stone moves with a speed of, say, eight while a smaller moves with a speed of four, then when they are united, the system will move with a speed less than eight; but the two stones when tied together make a stone larger than that which before moved with a speed of eight. Hence the heavier body moves with less speed than the lighter; an effect which is contrary to your supposition. Thus you see how, from your assumption that the heavier body moves more rapidly than the lighter one, I infer that the heavier body moves more slowly.

Field experiments take place in real situations

'Field experiments' contrast with laboratory experiments. They are often used in the social sciences, especially in economic analyses of education and health interventions. The natural setting of the experiment allows the field experiment to more closely represent the outcome in practice than would be gained in a laboratory environment. However, like natural experiments, field experiments suffer from the possibility of contamination: experimental conditions can be controlled with more precision and certainty in the laboratory.

A famous field experiment was conducted in 1747 by James Lind, who served as a surgeon in the British Royal Navy. He developed a cure for scurvy, from an experiment on 12 men from his ship. These men were divided into six pairs, giving each pair different additions to their basic diet for a period of 2 weeks. The treatments were all remedies that had been proposed at one time or another. They were: a quart of cider every day; twenty five guts (drops) of elixir vitriol (sulphuric acid) three times a day upon an empty stomach; one half-pint of seawater every day; a mixture of garlic, mustard and horseradish in a lump the size of a nutmeg; two spoonfuls of vinegar three times a day; two oranges and one lemon every day.

The men who had been given citrus fruits recovered dramatically within a week. One of them returned to duty after 6 days. The others experienced some improvement, but nothing was comparable to the citrus fruits, which were proved to be substantially superior to the other treatments. In this study his subjects' cases 'were as similar as I could have them', that is he provided strict entry requirements to reduce extraneous variation. The men were paired, which provided replication. From a modern perspective, the main thing that is missing is randomized allocation of subjects to treatments.

Observational studies are seen as less convincing evidence

'Observational studies' are similar to controlled experiments except that they lack probabilistic equivalency between groups. This means that study subjects are not placed into groups by the scientist, using random allocation or otherwise such as Lind, but are observed to be in a group through natural conditions. Observational studies arise in the area of medicine where, for ethical reasons, it is not possible to create a controlled group.

We may consider the results of observational studies as less convincing than results from controlled experiments. Observational studies are prone to forms of bias, such as selection bias and confounding. Researchers attempt to compensate for this with statistical methods. However, there are many situations where an experiment would not work. A good observational study may be better than a poorly controlled experiment.

The spread of cholera was minimized though observation and experiment

John Snow conducted a natural experiment on an unknowing London public. His genius showed in his meticulous and scientific way of conducting the natural experiment to prove his hypothesis that contaminated water is the vehicle for the cholera spread. In 1849, Londoners in Soho received drinking water supplies from two private water companies, Lambeth and Southwark companies. These companies drew water from the River Thames at a point named Battersea Fields where water was heavily contaminated with human sewage. Between 1845 and 1854, Lambeth Company changed its source of water collection to a point higher in the Thames where there was less pollution while Southwark Company continued to collect from the polluted source, Battersea Fields. After the source of collection was changed, a remarkable difference in number of cholera deaths between the two companies (5/1000 population in Southwark users versus 0.9/1000 population in Lambeth users) was observed. Snow found a decline in deaths in Lambeth customers while there was no fall in deaths of Southwark users who were still being supplied contaminated water from the same source.

Snow exploited this natural experiment and carried out a house to house survey of about 300,000 users of both companies and confirmed his hypothesis that cholera deaths were due to the contaminated water supplied by Southwark Company by comparing the death rates of both companies, by observing the reduction in mortality after Lambeth Company changed its source and by excluding other probable confounding factors. He considered all other causes that might confound his hypothesis and neutralized them. He had seen that no difference whatever existed, either in the houses or the people receiving water supply from the two water companies, or in any physical conditions with which they were surrounded.

Snow's endeavour, though exhaustive, is not an experiment in strict terms as he did not manipulate the event deliberately (Lambeth Company changed its source of collection by its own decision). This limitation does not reduce the greatness of his exploitation of a man-made disaster to reveal the mode of transmission of cholera before the cholera vibrio was discovered.

Summary

An experiment is a method of investigating causal relationships among variables with the results usually either rejecting or not the test hypothesis. Observational studies use naturally occurring groups, without direct manipulation by the epidemiologist to examine disease. Observational studies are seen as providing less-convincing evidence than experiments, but experimentation is not always possible, and epidemiologists must design studies that allow controlled conditions without resorting to random allocation of subjects.

Self-test questions

Q 1.5.1: According to Einstein, the development of western science is based on two achievements. What are they?

Q 1.5.2: A 'controlled experiment' compares the results obtained from _____ with _____?

Q 1.5.3: What is a natural experiment?

Q 1.5.4: When are observational studies most useful?

1.6   A Medical Sociological View

- Pre-requisite sections: None.
- Learning outcome: By the end of this section you should be able to describe what medical sociology is and how it can apply to epidemiology and its practice.

Medical sociology is the study of the constructs of health, illness and the way in which these ideas are measured. The measurement of ideas about health is common to both medical sociology and epidemiology. It is important to note that the idea of health is complex, meaning there exists a bigger idea made up of many smaller ideas. In both medical sociology and epidemiology, we need to think about how we measure these smaller ideas and in turn how these ideas are affected by what we measure.

Measurement of ideas can be thought of at varying levels. At one level we can think about the person and their actions. A broader example would be the hospital or indeed the process of medical education of the professionals working at the hospital, which can be important to health outcomes. At the broadest level would be the way a country organizes its healthcare system and the policies and outcomes associated with that organization which can greatly affect the health of the nation.

Let's go back to the basic level of idea measurement, that is a person's ideas and their actions. Take the example of the exchange of ideas between a client and his/her healthcare provider. Phil Brown notes in an interesting summary article, that when a client and health provider meet, it is more than just the language used, power differentials between them and the information exchanged (Brown, 1991). It is the professional, institutional, socio-cultural, political and economic factors that are also at work, shaping the outcomes and making a significant difference for the patient. Thus showing how the doctor's ideas about the health of the patient are affected by what he/she measures, the communications with the patient become important.

At a broader level of idea measurement, that of a national/regional issue, morbidity and mortality from acute diseases have been affected more by public health initiatives (for example sewers, clean water) and economic development (for example improving nutrition) than by medical treatments. This idea is an important area of interest for the formulation of public health policy. As we increasingly start to measure social constructs such as social support, social networks, class and race on disease incidence and spread of disease we can make a significant contribution to public health policy by using medical sociology to help guide epidemiology. It must always be borne in mind that interventions on a population may have other consequences that are not desirable (see Box 1.10).

How does this idea of measurement help an epidemiologist? Our aim is to look at the impact that existing traditions have on the individual and groups of individuals. Let's consider feminist sociology which grew out of the feminist movement and looks at how gender and power are interrelated. When feminist sociology first started, it was able to help ask questions in the broader field of medical sociology which helped to study the consequences of biases and poor practices for half the population, namely women. For example, counting the number of women having unnecessary hysterectomies or assessing the myth of the vaginal orgasm. Also by focusing on power differentials, a better study of the patient–health professional interaction was possible. A stronger focus on the outcomes of different practitioners, as found in women's health clinics also progressed the field (Brown, 1991).

Medical sociology concept 1: the sick role

Talcott Parsons defined the sick role as a temporary and sanctioned form of behaviour (Parsons, 1951). He noted that this illness construct had the benefit of giving an individual a reason for not completing their social responsibilities. The medical system provided a mechanism, altruistic at its base, for the individual to both be removed from their usual role of worker and then to return to their previous level of functioning through treatment. This seems to make sense but does it end there? If we simply accept this hypothesis and fail to test out our assumptions, then epidemiology will fail to progress.

What does this mean for patients in low socio-economic areas? When reaching low socio-economic, culturally and linguistically diverse communities, researchers often come up with difficulties in recruitment and losing individuals to follow-up. Engaging these patients requires strategies to address broader health issues such as affordability, ensuring cultural and language barriers are addressed through the use of culturally specific workers, the translation of materials and adapting programmes to the health beliefs and expectations of the target groups, improving health literacy and tailoring information and materials to accommodate different literacy levels and improving the communication skills of providers in order to address these barriers.

If we think just in terms of the sick role then it would be easy to justify labels such as 'waster' or 'slack' when describing groups that do not seem to benefit from existing healthcare arrangements. However, other organizational issues such as linking GPs, bilingual health workers, community health workers together with local community agencies do help to overcome the barriers to engagement of these hard to

---

Box 1.10. Individuals and populations

In 2007 the Australian federal government introduced the Northern Territory National Emergency Response, which implemented restrictions on alcohol in Aboriginal communities as a measure to curb the incidence of child sexual assault. It sounds good progress, lowering the incidence of damage to humans, but needs to be considered more widely.

Health is more than the absence of disease: it is a sense of wellbeing in many domains. There are other effects that this intervention may have. What about the effects on the society in which this intervention takes place? It limits a person's autonomy to act in the way they wish, even when they are not involved in child abuse. By taking control of the situation this way, the state is trying to remove the person's individual responsibility for the situation and damage caused. These are, surely, both fundamental human rights. What seems like a good idea needs to be thought through across all aspects of health, not just the absence of substance abuse. Such health interventions are often complicated situations containing many dilemmas.

---

reach groups. These successes ultimately call for further attention and study of the sick role as a concept in medical sociology and thus how it affects epidemiology.

Medical sociology concept 2: control of uncertainty in medicine

Most doctors are risk-averse whether it is a function of the increasingly litigious society in which they work, increasing expectations of the patients they treat or indeed as an outcome of the education they have received. Renee Fox notes, in her book *The Sociology of Medicine: A Participant Observer's View*, that emotional detachment is a means of medical students dealing with the uncertainties of their work (Fox, 1989). Doctors generally do not tolerate uncertainty and do not want anything bad to happen to their patients. Often the response is to over-test and over-treat in order to protect the patient. However this can also be seen as a means of protecting themselves.

Medical practitioners often feel judged – describing themselves as their harshest critics, however also judged by colleagues, patients and the healthcare system generally. The oath 'first do no harm' has been changed to 'do everything'. This relates to the increasing availability of tests often before their safety has been determined, and the cost–benefit ratio been calculated.

How has the training of medical practitioners influenced this? Robert Merton saw medical education as the training and socialization of the values of the medical profession generally (Merton *et al.*, 1957). Howard Becker put a greater emphasis on the medical student interpreting these values and the situation mediating the learning process (Becker *et al.*, 1961). It is important how detached and isolated the medical student group is from broader cultural influences, thereby affecting how these values are formed.

At a broader level, as a profession over the past two centuries we have seen the rise of the 'collegiate medical profession' - this is the body that determines who is qualified to practice medicine. Its emergence has come first out of the patronage system and/or a movement to increased state regulation as a means of dealing with the uncertainties associated with the practice of medicine. This seems to map closely to the emergence of the increasing use of hospital-based medicine. Medical treatment went from a doctor visiting a patient in their home to a patient visiting a hospital to seek treatment from a doctor.

Medical sociology allows us to see contemporary medical knowledge as not the outcome of a long process of improving our understanding of disease but more the triumph of one view, neither the first nor the last, of 'seeing' disease (Armstrong, 2009). The relationship between doctor and patient could be seen to be associated with changing systems of medical knowledge. The relationship between doctor and patient itself could be 'encoded', in the contemporary system of medical knowledge (Jewson, 2009). The emergence of pathological medicine, defined as medicine that searches for the cause of a disease, was not therefore the result of 'scientific progress' or unbiased outcome of applying the scientific method, but as the expression of a doctor–patient relationship with the doctor having power. Medical 'progress' can be seen as the result of the subjugation of the patient and a loss of their status as 'person' (Armstrong, 2009).

How does this happen? Sick men and women became first transposed into patients and thereafter into independent consumers of health care in market-based systems. People are treated first in their homes, then by examination in a clinic, then finally in labs where pathology and the genome rule and the social complexity and context is lost. It is important to note, how the health of the person is measured can be influential in how the patient is ultimately 'seen'.

Medical sociology concept 3: measurement and communication

Illness can be defined through a social lens, while disease itself seems to be the bio-medical manifestation of illness. Understanding the difference between these two concepts can influence how a patient interacts with his/her healthcare provider.

A consultation can be seen as a clinical event where a patient's physical, psychological and social problems are treated using medical care and advice. The patient consults with one or more of the healthcare team in the surgery/hospital, at the patient's home, in a co-operative, or over the telephone. The consultation is categorized as urgent or routine, initiated either by the patient or at the professional's request, in response to a need, or part of a formal review process. As epidemiology attempts to categorize behaviour, as we see above, medical sociology has a more holistic view.

An example of a consultation includes any of the following: a single visit for an acute illness, a follow-up after hospital admission, a medication review, a health promotion activity, a consultation for the management of a chronic disease, a consultation for screening, or for minor surgery.

Health professionals have traditionally used the 'consultation mapping' approach to structure the recording of a consultation. Developed in the classic text by Weed (1969) and known by the mnemonic SOAP (see Box 1.11), the format is used for consultations involving acute, minor, and chronic illnesses and is used by medical professionals in recording consultations in medical records (Weed, 1969; Lamberts *et al.*, 1993; Thom *et al.*, 2004).

The final part of the consultation is the action taken or proposed as a result of the assessment. The action taken can include advice, the issuing of a prescription, referral to other agencies and/or health professionals, further tests or investigations, or for a planned intent to consult with the patient again.

A patient's problems, whether physical, psychological, social or spiritual can be constructed as series of diagnoses or findings (Weed, 1969). In addition, a problem can be classified as either a sign or a symptom (Weed, 1969). In the consultation, signs relate to physiological findings and laboratory results, as they are objective in their indication of disease (Youngson, 1992). A symptom is subjective, suggesting a problem that cannot, by definition, be observed by others (Youngson, 1992). The

---

Box 1.11. Consultation mapping acronym

S - Subjective: What did the patient say?

O - Objective: What evidence of ill-health have I elicited?

A - Assessment: What do I make of the situation?

P - Plan: What am I going to do?

---

accurate measurement of a patient's problem is difficult. Different professionals measure the duration of a sign and/or symptom(s) from different time points. A measurement can be made from the symptom onset or alternatively from the date confirmed by a laboratory diagnosis (Wyatt, 1995). Psychological problems and their component symptoms are usually described with less definite aetiologies, with terms based on the sign related to the diagnosis (e.g. 'looks down' for patients with depression) (Willis, 1979).

As we can see, when a patient and health provider meet, the language used removes the patient from the consultation, the power differentials are maintained and the information exchanged is firstly defined by the medical fraternity and maintained during the recording of the event. The professional, institutional, socio-cultural, political, and economic factors shape the experience for the patient. For example, a non-compliant or non-concordant patient makes sense when power is considered. From a purely medical perspective, it makes no sense for a patient to not take their prescribed medication. However what may seem an illogical or irrational form of non-compliance with the good doctor's orders may be a well-thought-out plan on the part of the patient to avoid medical and social side-effects that impair the patient's personal and/or work life. These factors are more difficult to measure in terms of symptoms.

So, what does this mean? When a patient feels alienated by modern medicine or is defined as non-compliant or not concordant, there are many cultural aspects that might facilitate this experience. Sociologists might describe this as anomie where a society's norms and values break down for the individual (Durkheim, 1947). There are many similarities between these two experiences. Both have emerged with industrialization and would be experienced as similar feelings of disenchantment and unease. Beyond the scope of this section is to look at the international differences in health status and how interactions between countries help or hinder this. We could also consider the health labour force and its movement, and the provision of services across countries, the social control function of health services generally. This takes a very different view of health as a function of a capitalist system producing ill health and the existing social inequalities maintaining it through inequities in the provision of healthcare.

This could be seen as having potentially extreme outcomes and cause for alarm. A medicine based on pathology may mean that the humanity of the patient is lost. Modern medicine could represent the loss of a subjective identity which is part of human nature. However let's consider a thought experiment where the opposite may also be true. What if the objectification was not a negative process but a positive one? The 'object' of an analysable human body can be established through the very process of objectification. It can be hypothesized about, intervened with and modelled as to best ways to improve the experience of the person in terms of their health but also in terms of their humanness.

A new form of 'modern' identity, initially in an anatomical form, but then growing, and evolving into something new could be established. Greater choice and control in service delivery by people using a service could involve self-directed planning, self-directed funding and self-directed support. By increasing the focus on patients' rights and responsibilities, a better understanding of the problems patients experience in their dealings with the health system may be established. This could have implications for the research questions that are asked and the interventions that are implemented. Through shared decision making, open discussions about risk management and therefore sharing the uncertainty felt by both the patient and health professional, a new independent identity could be established.

Summary

As we increasingly start to measure social constructs that have been part of medical sociology for so long (for example social support, class and race) and their interactions with disease incidence we can begin to make a significant contribution to public health policy by using medical sociology to help guide epidemiology. We can look beyond the outcomes and engage people who may have been previously left behind and start to get the kind of reliable and valid outcomes that include the entire population.

Self-test questions

Q 1.6.1: What has affected mortality from acute diseases more than medical treatments?

Q 1.6.2: What does the mnemonic SOAP stand for?

Q 1.6.3: How did Parsons define the sick role?

Q 1.6.4: True or False - Medicine has at times been responsible for causing health problems as opposed to curing them?

Further Reading

Hennekens, C.H. (1987) *Epidemiology in Medicine*. Lippincott, Williams and Wilkins, London.

2 Cause and Effect

The identification of the determinants of health and disease is a primary goal for epidemiology. The sections in this chapter discuss and describe some of the important concepts of causality, which will help epidemiologists and students of statistical epidemiology to navigate the practical aspects of the science.

2.1 The Meaning of Causation

- Pre-requisite sections: 1.1, 1.2, 1.5.
- Learning outcome: By the end of this section you should be able to describe the meaning of causation and identify necessary and sufficient causes.

You may think to yourself that you know what 'causation' means; it is a straightforward word and a commonly used noun. Causation is defined as 'the action of causing' by the Oxford English Dictionary, which leads to the noun 'cause'. Cause is defined as 'a person or thing that produces an effect'. This also does not help us to disentangle how we identify a cause, as we must identify an effect to clarify a cause.

The knowledge of causation has implications for many people in many domains. Clinicians may have greater information on which to base treatment decisions. Scientists gain insight to allow development of novel therapies. Policy makers may act on known causes, such as banning smoking in public places, and these may influence education and personal choice. A growth in knowledge about causation has led, in part, to an increase in litigation.

Philosophical musings on causation

Many writers and philosophers have considered 'the action of causing'; David Hume, John Locke, John Stuart Mill and Bertrand Russell are among them. Hume laid the concepts down for this debate, clarifying that a cause is not an entity that can be observed; instead the observer sees the consequences of causation. John Locke stated that our internal world, or our imagining, is a representation of an object only if that object, and not a hallucination, caused it.

John Stuart Mill thought that causation was at the root of induction whereby any relationships between objects are discovered. Antecedent and consequent variables are used as part of the discussion and causation is the link between the two. Mill stated that the universal law of successive phenomena is the Law of Causation; every phenomenon is related, in a uniform manner, to some phenomenon that coexists with it. Bertrand Russell moved away from this deterministic view and took an inductive step by postulating natural laws governing the temporal and permanent nature of a variable, along a line or process.

Causes of a disease are critical to prevention

Philosophers have defined cause as the factor directly responsible for a given effect but this action is not directly observable. The cause of a disease is directly responsible for its incidence but is easily confused with elements that are correlated with, contribute to, or are associated with given effects. For example, sun exposure may be a cause of malignant melanoma, but various factors such as smoking and family history contribute to an individual's risk.

If we wish to prevent something, for example a disease, an accident, or a death, then it makes sense to identify the causes of this outcome. Epidemiologists also refer to the cause of an outcome as a risk factor, a determinant or an exposure. When we know what causes a disease we may be able to prevent the disease, we may be able to remove it or block its action. This is one of the main goals of public health and, as the adage goes, 'prevention is better than cure'. The effectiveness of this approach is encapsulated by one of the leading authorities on the prevention of disease, the Johns Hopkins Bloomberg School of Public Health, with their motto 'Protecting Health, Saving Lives – Millions at a Time'.

There are many notable examples of public health removing a cause of a disease. One of the most famous is the eradication of smallpox, which killed about 30% of sufferers and has been a major killer throughout history. Inoculation with the live smallpox virus prevented many outbreaks but led to a substantial mortality due to its inherent dangers. Jenner, in the 1790s, demonstrated smallpox could be prevented through vaccination with cowpox virus. The last naturally occurring cases of this killer disease were in Somalia in 1977, and there has not been a single case since then. There still exist stocks of the virus in laboratories, and controversy remains as to whether these should be destroyed forever. Many other causes of disease are not as straightforward to remove or prevent. For example, the breast cancer genes, BRCA1 and BRCA2 are inherited and lead to breast cancer. At the moment, inherited genetic mutations cannot be removed nor prevented; in this situation the knowledge allows screening and prophylactic measures.

We have an intuitive understanding of a cause

You may have thought that defining the meaning of causation was pointless and unnecessary. Have you ever thought how we, early in our lives, develop an intuitive understanding of causation? This skill allows us to navigate our environment safely, to know in advance the consequences of behaving in a certain way. How do we develop these skills? As a toddler, we develop a simple 'one cause leads to one event' model. For example, a toddler would watch a grown up using a light switch. They would see that the person clicked the switch and the light came on.

The toddler might think that the switch is the single cause of the light operating. Is the light switch the only cause for the light to come on? What about the light bulb or the electricity flowing correctly, which are other causes on the causal pathway? This is the same for epidemiology, where simplistic models are not sufficient to describe disease aetiology.

Hume developed a counterfactual approach to causation

How do we identify a cause? It is clear that a cause cannot be identified *per se*, but identified through its effects. Some of this falls into a realm of philosophy that has led to much discussion and debate. We do not propose to explore these here: we will introduce one approach to causation that has value for epidemiology.

We may assess whether a factor causes a disease by asking a simple question. Would the disease have happened anyway even if the factor were not present? Let's imagine we were to look at the causes of childhood leukaemia and were concerned about the use of mobile phones. In order to identify whether a mobile phone causes childhood leukaemia we would have to observe whether, in the same children at the same time, leukaemia occurred with the phone and did not occur without it. If the disease or outcome had happened even without the presence of the exposure, then we may deduce that the exposure we removed is not the only cause of that disease.

This is known as a counterfactual, it is counter to the facts, and does not occur in our real lives. David Hume, a Scottish philosopher, gave a definition of causation using a counterfactual argument as early as 1748: 'We may define a cause to be an object followed by another ... where, if the first object had not been, the second never had existed.'

A counterfactual is what would have happened if the cause had not been present. In the context of disease causation, a counterfactual situation is asking whether the outcome would have happened if the exposure had not been present, that is, if all of the other conditions were identical and the putative risk factor was removed. It is obviously not possible to observe a counterfactual. It is un-actualized, or counter to fact.

In Box 1.5 we explored a thought experiment using a counterfactual world. This is a strength of the thought experiment: counterfactual worlds can be imagined and used to identify causal relationships.

Study designs attempt to construct a counterfactual

In epidemiological study design the researcher attempts to create a version of the counterfactual population. It is not feasible to create a true counterfactual, but the scientist tries to create a close copy of one. This will differ depending on the type of design. A randomized controlled trial is the nearest design that can examine causation, as the control group represents the non-exposed counterfactual population. This allows comparison of an exposed group and non-exposed group. It is less clear how a case-control study represents the counterfactual, as the world without an exposure is not replicated. The comparison is a group of people without the outcome, not without the exposure as imagined in the counterfactual world.

Necessary and sufficient causes

Some types of cause may be 'necessary'; without a necessary cause the outcome, or effect, will not occur at all. Others may be 'sufficient', that is they, on their own, can produce an effect. If we return to our example where the toddler believes that the light switch causes the light to come on, the toddler will think that there is a one to one correspondence between the cause, which is the light switch, and effect, which is the light. In this example, the switch may or may not be necessary. There may be two light switches that control the same light and therefore one or other of the switches may not be a necessary cause of the light turning on. It is also clear that the switch is not a sufficient cause in that if the electricity in the house were turned off, the light switch would not work to turn the light on. We therefore say that the switch is not a sufficient cause.

Putting this into more structured terms for epidemiology, if an exposure is a necessary cause of an outcome, then the presence of that outcome implies the presence of the exposure. The presence of the exposure does not imply that the outcome will always occur. This is represented in Fig. 2.1 where it is not possible to have people who have the disease but do not have the necessary cause.

In contrast, for an exposure to be a sufficient cause of an outcome, then the presence of the exposure implies the presence of the outcome. However, there may be at least one more cause of the outcome and for this reason, the presence of the outcome does not necessarily imply the single exposure is present. This is depicted in Fig. 2.2.

It is very rare for a single sufficient cause to exist. Epidemiologists generally think about a series of minimal conditions or exposures that may lead to the development of disease. Referring back to the light bulb analogy, the light switch is not a single sufficient cause, but we could construct a set of conditions, such as the electricity being turned on, a light bulb being present, and so forth that might be sufficient to turn the light on.

Association is not necessarily causation

The concept of inference is an important central component of the statistical and scientific process. It is making a decision based on evidence, such as those you might make from observations. It may be that logic can also be used, although this is less likely to be applicable in epidemiology due to the complex nature of the evidence and the mechanisms involved.

		Disease	
		Present	Absent
Exposure	Present	✓	✓
	Absent		✓

Fig. 2.1. Representation of a necessary cause of an outcome.

		Disease	
		Present	Absent
Exposure	Present	✓	
	Absent	✓	✓

Fig. 2.2. Representation of a sufficient cause of an outcome.

One of the epidemiologist's jobs is to use observations and other forms of evidence to infer a cause of an outcome. This leads to a complicated situation: scientists and statisticians during their training are constantly reminded that, when there is an association between two variables A and B, this does not mean that there is a causal relationship. This may be due to random chance, or not knowing whether A causes B or B causes A. There may also be a third variable, C, where C causes both A and B and this leads to a statistical association between A and B.

This has led science, particularly medical sciences, into paying less attention to the concept of cause. We use language such as 'A implies B', 'A is associated with B' rather than 'A causes B'. As Pearl (2000) pointed out this has led scientists to not trusting themselves or others to explore causation, and even to avoid using the words: 'Causality is not mystical or metaphysical. It can be understood in terms of simple processes, and it can be expressed in a friendly mathematical language...' (Pearl, 2000).

Strength of an effect is the change in frequency of the outcome

An important piece of information about a putative risk factor is the impact it has on the frequency of disease. More precisely this is the change in disease frequency produced by introducing the factor into a population, because usually the disease will already exist in the population.

The strength of this effect is measured in absolute or relative terms. Absolute risk of disease, in simple terms, is the probability of disease and ranges between one, totally certain to happen, and zero, certain not to happen. This is different to measuring the strength of an effect in relative terms where the risk of the outcome is compared between the unexposed group and the exposed group. For example, the risk of disease in an exposed group of people may be three times the risk in a group of unexposed people.

Absolute measures of the strength of an effect are useful for planning public health and policy. They may also inform patients and the public to judge their risk against some other non-exposed group, however, they are less useful for aetiological epidemiology.

Induction and latent periods differ between exposures and outcomes

A 'latent period' is the time between exposure to a disease-causing agent and onset of disease. A disease may have incubated but remains latent, or dormant, within the body. For example, the time between exposure to HIV infection and the onset of AIDS can be years. This should be distinguished from incubation, which is the difference in time between a pathogen entering the body and when first symptoms appear.

The 'induction' period is the time between the end of the final component on the causal pathway and initiation of the disease. It is often used in laboratory or clinical sciences to define the interval between an initial injection of an antigen and the appearance of antibodies in the blood. The induction period may range between many years, for example hypertension leading to heart muscle thickening, and nanoseconds, for example a DNA strand breaks by ultraviolet radiation.

Researchers may have some difficulty defining these time points. For example, hepatitis C is an infectious disease affecting the liver, caused by the hepatitis C virus (HCV). Symptoms may include jaundice, fatigue, flu-like symptoms, and dark urine, but it may be asymptomatic for many years with the infection leading to scarring and damage of the liver. This makes defining the true time at which disease onsets difficult, but you may be able to use biomarkers such as a positive HCV RNA level and a positive HCV antibody test to determine these two points.

Initiator and promoter

'Initiator' and 'promoter' are terms used to describe exposures for the development of chronic disease, where the disease has multiple stages in its development. The initiator is the first exposure or cause that will eventually lead to the outcome. The promoters are all subsequent causes on the causal pathway that increase expression of the disease in the population.

For example, coronary heart disease is a multi-factorial, multistage disorder, which has both environmental and genetic factors. Is a gene the initiator or first cause or does it have a promoter role in the disease? Some laboratory-based specialties, such as molecular epidemiology have a saying that a genetic predisposition for a disease 'loads the gun' and an environmental factor 'pulls the trigger'. The genetic makeup of the individual may be considered an initiator, but as you can see it is not sufficient to cause the disease.

Summary

If we wish to prevent something, a disease, an accident, or a death, then it makes sense to identify the causes of this outcome. Policy makers may act on known causes, such as banning smoking in public places, and these may impact on education and personal choice. We need to answer the question, would the disease have happened anyway even if the factor were not present?

Self-test questions

Q 2.1.1: What can we do to prevent illness when we know its cause?

Q 2.1.2: Define a counterfactual.

Q 2.1.3: What research design most closely mirrors the counterfactual approach?
A A randomized controlled trial
B A case-control study
C An ecological study
D Anecdote

Q 2.1.4: Is the latent period of a disease

A Time from birth to disease onset?

B Time from exposure to a cause to onset of disease?

C Time from onset of disease to onset of symptoms?

2.2 Models of Causation

- Pre-requisite sections: 2.1.
- By the end of this section, you should be able to describe methods for investigating causation.

How do you analyse and infer causation? This is a challenge for epidemiology and because of this epidemiologists have developed many ways to model causation. Each method has good aspects and bad, and we do not have one perfect method. Indeed, it is not uncommon for scientists to use a number of methods. We will describe multiple methods and provide examples to assist the reader in identifying which may be most applicable to different research fields.

Method 0: 'three times is true'

An interesting facet of human nature is that when something is identified three times it is sometimes considered a 'true fact'. Lewis Carroll used this in a poem about a crew from a ship hunting for a fictional character, the Snark (see Box 2.1). The leader of the crew, the Bellman, has stated a case three times and therefore, he believes the crew should consider this true. This is known as the Bellman's fallacy.

This is a nonsensical example, but there have been unfortunate incidents of this in real life. Dr Roy Meadow, a British paediatrician, has views on cot death that were eventually discredited, but before this his views had great implications on peoples' lives.

Meadow's cot death theory was that one infant death was a tragedy, two in the same family was suspicious and three was murder (Watkins, 2000). This explanation has since been rejected in UK and US courts but demonstrates how a layperson may think they understand how to calculate the probability of an event (see Box 2.2).

Box 2.1. The hunting of the Snark by Lewis Carroll (1876)

(Part 1) The landing

'Just the place for a Snark!' the Bellman cried,
As he landed his crew with care;
Supporting each man on the top of the tide
By a finger entwined in his hair.
'Just the place for a Snark!;
I have said it twice: That alone should encourage the crew.
Just the place for a Snark!;
I have said it thrice: What I tell you three times is true.'

> **Box 2.2. Prosecutor's fallacy**
>
> Meadow's cot death theory stated that the chance of three cot deaths occurring in a single family was so small that it is most likely to be murder unless proven otherwise. It is a classic prosecutor's fallacy.
>
> A fallacy is an incorrect idea, named after the simple, but incorrect, method of calculating the probability of an event. Meadow took the cube of the probability of having a cot death in a family, and said this was so rare that it is not possible for it to be by chance. However, in a case where babies have already died, this doesn't apply. The simple calculation done by Meadows is the probability of choosing a family at random and finding that three cot deaths have occurred in that family, but what we need is to estimate the probability that they died of natural causes against the probability they were killed. Using this calculation, it turns out to be much more likely they died of natural causes.
>
> This is why it is essential for a statistician to be an expert witness in such a case, rather than relying on the evidence from a clinically trained doctor. Humans are very good at estimating distance and angles, but poor when it comes to probability theory.

Method 1: Koch's postulates

Koch's postulates, formulated by Robert Koch and Friedrich Loeffler in 1884, are four criteria designed to establish that a disease is caused by a microorganism:

1. The microorganism must be found in all organisms suffering from the disease, but should not be found in healthy organisms.
2. The microorganism must be able to be isolated from a diseased organism and grown in culture.
3. The microorganism, grown in culture, should cause disease when introduced into a healthy organism.
4. The microorganism must be re-isolated from the organism that the cultured microorganism was introduced to and identified as being identical to the original microorganism.

Koch applied these postulates to establish the aetiology of anthrax and tuberculosis. The first of these, known as the universalist requirement, was dropped by Koch as there are many diseases, particularly viral diseases, that have carriers of the microorganisms but the carriers do not have the disease. These asymptomatic carriers exist in cholera and typhoid fever for example.

The second postulate may also be suspended, as we may not be able to culture the microorganism, due to human's inability to grow the microorganism artificially rather than proof that it is not a causative agent of a disease. The third postulate may also be called into question. Many microorganisms may be introduced into a host organism and only a small proportion of hosts go on to develop the disease. This is the case for polio, where the poliovirus is beyond doubt the cause of the disease, but only a proportion of exposed humans develop polio. This is due to other factors such as the host's immune system.

With these caveats in mind Koch's postulates may be useful as a causal model for infectious disease, but they remain less useful for disease from other agents.

Method 2: find or invent a counterfactual world

The counterfactual approach to assessing cause asks 'What would have happened if this putative causative agent were not present?' These are 'unactualized possibilities' and are 'conceived of' events, thought up by the researcher.

They are not objectifiable in themselves, and are mind-made (Rescher, 1979) or in other words exist in the realm of the 'could be' but 'aren't'. Philosophers have visualized them occurring in alternative worlds and authors have made use of this editorial device to great effect. A great example is the novel *The Plot Against America* by Philip Roth (2004) which is an alternate history of the United States where Franklin Delano Roosevelt is defeated in the election of 1940 by Charles Lindbergh and the Nazis win the Second World War. This approach is not likely to provide a means to identify a cause. Using a thought experiment may achieve this, whilst some epidemiology study designs attempt to replicate a counterfactual.

Method 3: randomized controlled trial

The best real-life scientific approach we have is a randomized controlled trial (RCT). An RCT is a scientific experiment set up to determine how useful an intervention may be in the laboratory or in the field. An RCT can be used to test drugs, a service delivery model or indeed a product like a mobile phone. The random allocation of patients to different interventions (treatments or conditions) is the key.

The advantages of such an approach are that it provides good evidence for causality, and it removes many biases that appear in observational study designs. Unfortunately RCTs are expensive and often entirely inappropriate in many situations. For example, were we interested in the possible effects of mobile phones to primary school children, is it ethical to give some children a mobile phone and others not?

Method 4: synthesize the evidence

One of the roles for epidemiology is to put together, and to synthesize, the evidence that has been discovered. The aim is to use strategies that give other researchers the knowledge to separate causal from non-causal associations. We do this by using inductive reasoning of sufficient strength and rigour to be successful.

Meta-analysis is one of the ways that has been developed to combine the statistical information from multiple similar studies and provides statistical tests for the overall results. These can be effect sizes such as relative risks or probability from statistical tests. This may also be incorporated into a systematic review of the literature and using experts to examine the evidence. Epidemiologists looking to synthesize information must be aware that many statistical tests cannot be given a causal meaning.

Method 5: Hill's roadmap

Austin Bradford Hill, an eminent epidemiologist, developed a series of criteria for assessing a causal agent for a disease (Hill, 1965). These are:

1. Strength. The stronger the association between a proposed causal factor and an outcome, the less likely this may be explained by confounding. However, a weak association may still demonstrate a causal association.

2. Consistency. When multiple studies, in different circumstances, lead to the same conclusions this provides evidence for a causal relationship. This is central to the concept of replication when adhering to scientific method.

3. Specificity. The causative factor is linked to a specific causal mechanism.

4. Temporality. Exposure precedes disease by a reasonable amount of time. This is a standard and important facet of causality.

5. Biological gradient. Does an increasing amount of exposure increase the risk? If a dose–response relationship is present, there is strong evidence for a causal relationship. When a dose–response relationship is absent a causal relationship is not ruled out, as a threshold may exist above which a relationship may develop.

6. Plausibility. Plausible mechanism may be important, even in the face of known biological or epidemiological evidence, but equally all that is plausible is not always true.

7. Coherence. All facts stick together to form a coherent whole. Laboratory evidence supporting an association would underline a causal conclusion and help identify a causal agent. However, the absence of laboratory knowledge would not be suggestive of a non-causal explanation.

8. Experimental. Imagine standing on the shoulders of giants. A causal interpretation of an association from a non-experimental study can be supported if a randomized prevention confirmed the finding.

9. Analogy. Similarities among things that are otherwise different. This is a weak form of evidence.

Some epidemiological studies have used these criteria. They were designed to provide a systematic approach to synthesizing evidence with expert opinion.

Method 6: causal component model

The causal component model was developed by Rothman to allow epidemiologists to visualize the factors that were sufficient to cause a disease. Figure 2.3a gives, for

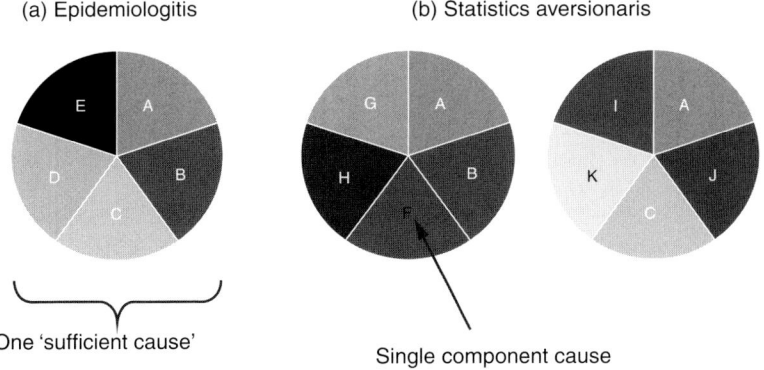

Fig. 2.3. Causal components model.

a hypothetical disease, a single sufficient causal component model. The exposures A, B, C, D and E are necessary and, combined, are sufficient to develop the disease.

In Fig. 2.3b there are two sets of causal components sufficient to cause the disease. One of these, component A, is present for both sets of cause. This, therefore, is a necessary cause as neither of the two models of cause could operate without this one component.

Method 7: causal graphs

Causal graphs, known as directed acyclic graphs (DAGs), are a fairly new domain for epidemiology. These models began in artificial intelligence systems and have been pioneered by a few notable epidemiologists. The graphs depict the variables, or nodes, that go into a system that eventually leads to an outcome or disease. A variable, known as a node, is represented on a figure. When a variable causes another variable, an arrow is drawn with the arrow pointing from the causal variable towards the effect. This is done for all of the variables represented on the DAG.

These models can be complex, allowing the epidemiologist to place a structure on the relationships between the entities within the system. The models can then be used to examine sufficient sets of causal components, confounding, and methods to intervene to prevent an outcome.

Summary

There is no single, perfect, method to model the causal relationships between variables. Many scientists have developed many approaches to this, beginning with Koch's postulates which are specific to infectious pathogens and their relationship to disease. It is common for an epidemiologist to use many approaches, including systematic reviews, meta-analysis and causal diagrams. Directed acyclic graphs are becoming a more widespread tool for examining cause.

Self-test questions

Q 2.2.1: Which of these are useful models of causation (none, one or more than one)?
A Rothman's causal components model
B Counterfactual worlds
C Directed acyclic graphs
D Randomized controlled trials

Q 2.2.2: Why is a randomized controlled trial the best approach we have, in practice, to evaluate causal links?

Q 2.2.3: Which of these groups represents a counterfactual world?
A Cases of disease not given a new drug in a trial of that new drug

B Cases of disease given the new drug in a trial of that new drug
C People without a disease to be compared in their smoking habits to people with a disease under investigation
D People without a disease who were not exposed to a water contaminant

2.3 Visualizing Cause

- Pre-requisite sections: 2.1, 2.2.
- Learning outcome: By the end of this section you should be able to describe the terms used in causal diagrams, construct simple diagrams and identify the strengths and weaknesses of visualizing cause in this way.

Researchers often want to discover causative links, such as whether a certain exposure causes a disease. Much of the aetiological research that is conducted is not experimental but is based on observational research. Experimental research is one of the best ways to detect causal relationships; however, many research situations cannot be addressed using experiments conducted on human beings.

Scientists have not been dissuaded from examining causal relationships using observational data. Hume, and many other philosophers, have discussed how it is not possible to see a cause, you can only see the consequences of a cause. At the forefront of research to visualize a causal mechanism are diagrams used by scientists called directed acyclic graphs (DAGs).

Constructing causal diagrams is intuitive

Figure 2.4 shows a simple DAG, which depicts the variables, known as nodes, or vertices, which go into a system that eventually leads to an outcome or disease. Each node is represented by a word written on the figure. When there is a causal relationship between two nodes, this is depicted by a line connecting each node, called an arc or edge or line. The arcs are directed, which means they have an arrowhead on one side only. This shows that when an exposure points at an outcome that the exposure causes that outcome.

When Sir Richard Doll was investigating lung cancer due to smoking, he would have constructed a DAG with an arrow from the node 'smokes tobacco' to the node 'lung cancer'. This DAG would be constructed from knowledge from previous robust empirical studies, understanding from a firm grasp of the functional biological, social or clinical relationships between variables or, as was the case for Doll, speculation. The nodes are often arranged in temporal order, with the earliest variables on the left of the diagram and the latest on the right. This is

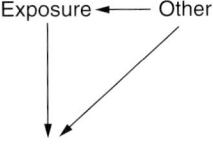

Fig. 2.4. A simple directed acyclic graph (DAG).

not mandatory, but can help when deciding which of two closely related variables precedes the other and acts as its cause.

The DAG allows the scientist to visualize the causal relationships in a system in an intuitive way. It seems natural to use an arrow to describe the direction of an effect and this is the basis of causal diagrams. Causal diagrams entered the mainstream scientific community following the publication of Pearl's book (Pearl, 2000). They allow the scientist to think clearly about how exposure, disease and potential confounder variables are related to each other. Causal diagrams also allow the author to communicate various inter-relationships to the reader, to indicate which variables were important to measure, and to inform the statistical modelling process. This last point is particularly useful in the identification of competing exposures and confounders.

Paths link variables with arrows

A path, or route, is the sequence of arcs connecting two or more nodes, thus X→Y→Z is the path connecting the nodes X and Z. Directed graphs are where every arc has only one arrow, indicating that no variable can be simultaneously the cause and effect of another. A direct or causal path is one where the arcs all follow in the direction of causality.

A confounder may be identified by being on a 'backdoor path' between an outcome and a putative risk factor. A backdoor path is where one exits a node along an arc pointing into it, against the causal direction, to another node across any number of arcs pointing in either direction. For example, a backdoor path exists between X and Z via Y when X→Y→Z.

A node becomes a 'collider' where both arcs of the path entering and leaving the node have arrows pointing into it. For example, Y is a collider on the X to Z path where X→Y←Z. A path is blocked if it contains at least one collider. Box 2.3 gives many other terms used in constructing DAGs.

A DAG must not have a circuit of arcs

A directed acyclic graph occurs if no directed path forms a closed loop, reflecting the fact that no variable can cause itself. All arcs in a DAG reflect *a priori* assumptions about cause and effect in a specific context, some based on firm knowledge and understanding of the actual or likely relationships between variables, others based on speculative hypotheses (including the specific relationships examined in the analyses). These assumptions cannot be inferred empirically from data on which the analyses will be conducted, but must be drawn from previous robust empirical studies or from a firm understanding of the functional biological, social and clinical relationships between the variables involved.

Nodes and arcs are based on prior knowledge

The knowledge of the nodes and their causal relationships is crucial for developing an accurate DAG as the basis on which suitable statistical analyses can then be designed

Box 2.3. Glossary of terms for causal diagrams

ancestor	a variable that causes another variable in a direct path
arc	a line with one arrow that connects two nodes
backdoor path	a path that goes against the direction of the first single headed arrow on the path, but can then follow or oppose the direction of any subsequent single headed arrows
blocked path	a path that contains at least one collider
causal path	a path that follows the direction of the single headed arrows: a direct path
child	a variable that is directly affected by another variable
collider	a variable that a path enters and exits via arrowheads
descendant	a variable that is caused by one or more preceding variables in a direct path
direct path	a path that follows the direction of the single headed arrows: a causal path
directed arc	an arrow between two nodes that indicates prior knowledge, understanding or assumption of cause
edge	*see* arc
line	*see* arc
node	a point within the diagram which denotes a variable, such as the (key) exposure variable of interest, the (key) outcome (of interest) or another covariate
non-directed arc	an arc without arrowheads that demonstrates that two variables are associated with one another (even though one does not cause the other) because both have a cause in common. Non-directed arcs may be found on a blocked or unblocked path
parent	a variable that directly affects another variable
path	an unbroken route between adjacent nodes, in either direction
route	*see* path
unblocked path	a path that does not contain a collider
vertex	*see* node

(Tu *et al.*, 2004; Weinberg, 2005). DAGs may be used to identify the most appropriate statistical analyses for any given set of measured variables. They will reduce the likelihood that these are subject to confounding and they help others to critique, reinterpret and where possible repeat and improve on the analyses conducted. Identification of the most appropriate statistical analyses and replication are the core strengths of using DAGs to design the analysis of data from non-experimental studies.

A potential limitation of DAGs is that, despite the potential for visual complexity, particularly of DAGs with more than a handful of nodes, they can be an oversimplification of the causal relationships between variables. For example, a causal diagram does not indicate whether an effect is harmful or protective or whether effect modification is occurring or not (Hernan *et al.*, 2004). A causal diagram cannot identify whether a cause is sufficient or necessary (Rothman, 1976). Yet, one of the key strengths of such diagrams is that they enable the researcher to think clearly and logically about the research question at hand, and to make explicit any assumptions made about the presumed relationships between pairs of variables. A visual summary can then be used as an aid to communicate these inter-relationships to other researchers. This can explicitly identify, for example, if important variables or relationships are missing from or misrepresented in the diagram or, indeed, whether any of the presumed relationships are contentious.

Speculative nature of DAGs

In most research studies the causal pathways described and summarized within causal diagrams are not 'proven' causal relationships, but are based on evidence from whatever previous studies are available. Proof in this sense is more a philosophical concept. The pathways included in the diagrams are therefore often based on empirical findings, which may not themselves be definitive.

The ways in which causal pathways can be conceptualized influence the extent to which different causal diagrams can be drawn for the same variables. These also may limit the extent to which different diagrams might be useful for generating robust evidence of causality between two variables. Despite this, DAGs force researchers to make explicit their assumptions about the relationships between pairs of variables, whether or not these assumptions prove to be correct.

Strengths and weaknesses of causal diagrams

One of the main strengths in using causal diagrams in epidemiological analyses of data from non-experimental studies is that it enables researchers to think clearly and logically about the potential causal relationships. At the same time, causal diagrams then allow researchers to communicate the causal assumptions they have made concerning these inter-relationships to other researchers using a structured approach.

DAGs enable the identification of variables that are important to measure in a prospective research study. DAGs also improve the efficiency of data collection and the efficiency of statistical analyses by avoiding the unnecessary measurement or inclusion of variables that are irrelevant to the study and analyses. DAGs can be used to identify confounding and confounders in a systematic way, and by helping researchers to identify these objectively and explicitly, DAGs can help to reduce bias and advance debate.

A weakness with DAGs is that with increasing numbers of highly inter-related variables they can very rapidly become visually complex to read. Moreover, as with all causal models, DAGs are only as good as the assumptions, knowledge and hypotheses on which they are based. In particular, DAGs may be based on a set of assumptions that are wrong because of incorrect understanding of hypotheses.

Summary

Directed acyclic graphs (DAGs) have great potential utility in epidemiological analyses of data from non-experimental studies, not least because they encourage researchers to formally structure presumed and predicted causal pathways. These causal diagrams are essentially intuitive to construct but nonetheless require considered thought. As with all models, careful interpretation is imperative. With satisfactory construction they can be used to identify sufficient sets of confounders which will greatly advance analytical modelling strategies and subsequent critique, testing and re-modelling by other researchers.

Self-test question

Q 2.3.1: A variable is represented as a
A node?
B line?
C arc?
D confounder?

Further Reading

Cochran, G.M., Ewald, P.W., Cochran, K.D. (2000) Infectious causation of disease: An evolutionary perspective. *Perspectives in Biology and Medicine*, 43, 3 Spring 2000, 406–449.

3   An Epidemiologist's Toolkit

The epidemiologist must use the correct tools to address the research questions that need answering. There are many different approaches that may be taken, and each has its own disadvantages and advantages. This section gives detail about each of the main approaches, and discusses the most appropriate situations that these may be used in. An overarching example, cervical cancer, is used throughout to highlight the way the cause of this disease has been discovered and prevented.

3.1   A Problem for Epidemiology

- Pre-requisite sections: 1.1, 1.3, 2.1.
- Learning outcome: By the end of the section you should be able to describe an example of a disease that needs investigating.

There are many success stories created by the work of science, and epidemiology, leading to the implementation of public health measures to improve people's lives. For example, we now understand the risks of excessive sun exposure for malignant melanoma, and the role that tobacco smoking plays in the development of lung cancer.

In Chapter 3 we focus on the major types of epidemiological study design. Many of these will be accompanied by the practical difficulties in implementing the design and the potential for bias. The advantages and disadvantages inherent in each design will be discussed.

Study designs are illustrated with cervical cancer research

Each section on study design will use an overarching example of a disease that is a major killer, but through many years of research is now becoming preventable. This disease is cancer of the cervix. The cervix is the opening (cervix means 'neck' in Latin) of the uterus. Cancer of the cervix has been recognized for two millennia, with Hippocrates describing the disease in 400 BCE (Gasparini and Panatto, 2009). This must be the first stage in finding a preventative measure. According to figures from the World Health Organization for 2010, cancer of the cervix is diagnosed in 510,000 women each year. Of these it kills 288,000. It is the second most common death from cancer in women after breast cancer, amounting to approximately 10% of all cancers.

Progress in early detection

The incidence of cervical cancer in England and Wales fell by 42% in a little under 10 years. Why was this? A cervical screening programme was introduced that, during a 2-year period (1990–1992), led to a 25% decrease in the incidence of cervical cancer for women younger than 70. The increased uptake of the cervical screening programme that occurred during this time led to greatly increased detection. In 1995 there were 10.4 newly diagnosed cases of cervical cancer per 100,000 women. By the end of the decade this had fallen to 9.3 per 100,000 women. Cervical screening itself now saves at least 1300 lives per year in the UK. For the first time death rates from cervical cancer are below 1000 per year in England; in 2002, 927 deaths from cervical cancer were registered. But there remains room for improvement.

At present, women should first be called for screening at age 25 as invasive cancer is rare in women younger than 25. Changes in the cervix are common before 25 and therefore younger women may get an abnormal result when there is nothing wrong. These false positive results lead to unnecessary investigations and treatments. For women aged 25 to 49 it is recommended they attend three-yearly and women aged 50 to 64 should attend five-yearly.

In terms of risk, women who have had many sexual partners, or whose partners have had many partners, are more at risk of developing cervical cancer. Women who smoke are about twice as likely to develop cervical cancer as non-smokers while women who take immunosuppressant drugs are more at risk of developing cervical cancer.

The screening process

One of the screening methods, called liquid-based cytology, involves preparing cervical samples for examination in a laboratory. A sample of cervical cells is taken using a brush which is either broken off into a small glass vial containing preservative fluid, or the head is rinsed directly into the preservative fluid in the vial and then disposed of. Liquid-based cytology reduces the number of inadequate cervical tests as this was an issue with previous types of testing.

The diagnosis process

Following a positive screen, a low-powered microscope known as a colposcope is used to examine the cervix and assess the severity of any problem. Colposcopy allows a biopsy to be taken from the cervix under direct vision. If the histological diagnosis indicates grade 2 or grade 3, known as CIN 2 or 3, the affected part of the cervix should be removed or destroyed. For women with CIN 1, monitoring is best as it often disappears without treatment. If there are problems in assessment, for example if the abnormal area cannot be seen with a colposcope, the woman may need a cone biopsy.

There are two main types of treatment

The abnormal cells can be cut away using loop diathermy or the abnormal cells can be destroyed using laser ablation or cold coagulation. The treatment aims to preserve fertility. Surgery is the main form of treatment for the few women who have cancer, while radiotherapy and chemotherapy may be used.

The disease seriously affects developing countries, where 80% of the diagnoses are made. Pre-invasive cervical neoplasia 'continues at epidemic proportions' (Rubin, 2001). Incidence of cervical cancer has two peaks occurring at ages thirty-five years and sixty-four years.

Summary

Despite the major advances in detection, treatment and care, the goal should be to prevent the disease in the first place. The fight to prevent cervical cancer provides an excellent example of epidemiology at work. It demonstrates the importance of the various methods to chip away at the prevention conundrum. It is a story of characters, scientists, and patients, and culminates in the Nobel Prize for Physiology or Medicine in 2008. Some of these characters will have made decisions (see Box 3.1), but the hope is that epidemiology has managed to prevent a killer disease.

Self-test question

Q 3.1.1: What are the possible reasons that cervical cancer incidence fell?

3.2 Anecdote

- Pre-requisite sections: 1.2, 1.4, 2.1, 3.1.
- Learning outcome: By the end of the section you should be able to understand the limitations of anecdote to inform science and epidemiology.

Anecdote describes anything spoken, or written down, that reports an interesting observation. In common usage, it may be the basis for a joke or a witty remark, or an

---

Box 3.1. Objective beliefs

The concept of objectivity is not as straightforward as it may at first seem. Science is about measuring things correctly, and, as scientists, we do our best to uphold that tradition. The definition of objectivity, however, is 'the perception of things'. This is therefore in fact subjective as all things measured are perceived. This affects scientists' ability to measure things perfectly. Even though epidemiologists behave ethically, there are a number of routes to biased data collection, analysis and reporting of results for all scientists. One such route is when a scientist has a favourite 'pet' hypothesis, and particularly when a hypothesis is named after a person. There have been examples where an epidemiologist ignores data and results that do not support, or even that reject, their hypothesis. It doesn't need to be consciously done and it is clear that it is sometimes unconscious, but either way some decisions may lead to biased findings.

---

incident in someone's life. In clinical medicine and epidemiology, it often relates to an observation of a new disease, or observation that an environmental factor may be involved in causing a disease. Medicine has a formalized system of anecdote, known as the case series.

Anecdote and storytelling generally have an important role to play in society. As author Phillip Pullman pointed out, stories are powerful tools for humans: 'We don't need lists of rights and wrongs, tables of do's and don'ts: we need books, time, and silence. 'Thou shalt not' is soon forgotten, but 'Once upon a time' lasts forever.' (Phillip Pullman, in his acceptance speech for the 1996 Carnegie Medal).

Anecdote is used carefully in science

Anecdote is defined as a short account of an amusing or interesting event and is usually connected with a particular person. It is from the Greek meaning 'things unpublished', which goes against one of the main activities of science which is to publish findings. This allows other scientists to review the findings and try to replicate them.

A medically centred anecdote may be a story relating to an individual's experience with their disease or symptoms. The reader of an anecdote may find it interesting, or they may 'believe' the story as it in some way relates to their values or experiences. The word 'story' has different meaning and understandings for different people. Humans are keen to hear or read a story, we are interpreting beings and we enjoy seeking meaning in other people's experiences. We try to give meanings to our own experiences throughout our lives.

Scientists are deeply suspicious of anecdote. However humans are social storytelling animals – we instinctively learn by the experience of others. From an evolutionary perspective when my friend ate that plant with the bright red berries and then became ill I learnt a lesson: don't eat from that plant. It is much quicker and easier to avoid the plant with the red berries rather than conduct double blinded experiments to see if it really was the plant that made your friend sick or something else. These are quick ways to navigate our environment.

Anecdote in clinical medicine

We have evolved to deal with all of the data we are confronted with. The primary weakness of anecdote is that they are not controlled. Other problems include

- Regression to the mean is the statistical phenomenon whereby an extreme result is more likely followed by a result closer to the average. Often diseases have variable symptoms. Therefore when you seek out a treatment when the symptoms are severe, by chance this is likely followed by a period when the symptoms are not as severe.
- Most illnesses are self-limiting, most ailments get better or improve on their own, and most treatments will be followed by symptom resolution even if the treatment has no effect.

- Multiple treatments will often be tried by people for a disease making it near impossible to tell which treatment worked.
- Reporting bias may be caused because people who die of a disease are not around to give their anecdotes.
- Confirmation bias as people tend to seek out and remember information that confirms what we already believe, and forget or explain away evidence against it.
- Vague outcome measures. Science uses objective outcome measures while subjective symptoms do not make good outcome measures.
- Fallibility of memory as people may, from their memory, exaggerate the severity of symptoms prior to treatment, amend the timeline of events so that improvement began very soon after a treatment and forget other treatments.

Anecdote in epidemiology

Anecdote does not generally play an important role in epidemiological research as it is not perceived as part of the scientific method. However, the initial stage in the scientific method requires the scientist to make observations. These observations may fall under the banner of anecdote.

There are many reasons to publish anecdotes, including describing a newly recognized adverse reaction or interaction, generating hypotheses, testing hypotheses, demonstrating diagnostic techniques, elucidating mechanisms, elucidating or suggesting methods of management, educating and as the basis for systematic review. The science community does not see anecdote, when reported by non-scientists, as valid. It is disingenuous to maintain this position for all anecdotes. An example of where anecdote has been really important is in the first recognized cases of acquired immunodeficiency syndrome (AIDS) that occurred in the United States of America in the early 1980s. A number of homosexual men in New York and San Francisco began to develop rare opportunistic infections and cancers that seemed stubbornly resistant to any treatment. At this time, AIDS did not yet have a name, but it quickly became obvious that all the men were suffering from a common syndrome.

A syndrome is the association of several clinically recognizable features: signs which are occurrences observed by another person and symptoms which are reported by the patient that occur together. The presence of one feature alerts the clinician or researcher to the presence of the other parts of the syndrome. In recent decades, the term has been used outside medicine to refer to a combination of phenomena seen in association. For example, AIDS is a syndrome that is based on evidence of human immunodeficiency virus (HIV) infection and the development of one or more of a list of opportunistic infections or malignancies for which there is no other explanation, for example the most common, which account for up to 80% of the defined AIDS cases, are *Pneumocystis carinii* pneumonia and Kaposi's sarcoma.

When reporting anecdote, as with other types of research it is important to be consistent. Reporting cases uniformly facilitates direct comparisons of individual reports and detailed information allows the reader to obtain the information. Standardized reporting of anecdote would also facilitate systematic review of suspected reactions (Aronson, 2003).

Anecdote causes controversy

With the advent of easily accessible litigation in society there seems to have been a growth in the observation that '… there are X cases of disease Y in my neighbourhood …'. These reports of disease may not seem relevant to medical research but, on occasion, they have played an important role in epidemiology and clinical science. Returning to the AIDS example, one of the difficult situations with the anecdote was that the disease was first recognized only in homosexual men. This was potentially damaging, and continues to play a role in the global thinking on HIV/AIDS prevention and treatment.

The media are often keen to report anecdote, placing 'human interest' above scientific validity. The public often notice patterns in situations, where none may really exist. However, even in these cases it is possible that the media reporting of observations may be important for public health. For example, in the early 1980s Yorkshire Television broadcast a programme called *Windscale: The Nuclear Laundry* which was about a number of cases of leukaemia and lymphoma in Seascale, the village near to the nuclear installation of Windscale, later known as Sellafield. These anecdotes were comprehensively investigated and led to the setting up of monitoring systems in the United Kingdom, such as SAHSU (www.sahsu.org).

Anecdote may drive research hypotheses

Some anecdotes, given time, have been shown to be correct, generating a useful hypothesis for science to test. Box 3.2 reports on a famous anecdote on the low risk of cervical cancer in nuns. With hindsight, this anecdote has had some basis in the truth.

Did this anecdote help epidemiology? Given a large research effort, with the benefit of hindsight we now accept that a sexually transmitted infection, human papillomavirus (HPV), causes cervical cancer. The anecdote was helpful in providing a potential avenue for risk investigation.

Anecdote cannot be tested using scientific method

The main problem with using anecdote as scientific evidence is that it is not collected in an appropriate manner. For example, it is common for anecdote to report that a person, exposed to a known risk factor, did not contract the disease associated with that risk factor. This point is illustrated with an example in Box 3.3.

Epidemiology does not provide a definitive answer for an individual, it states the overall risk for a person, which is rarely, if ever, 100%. These anecdotes often illustrate the exceptions to the risk, but they do not disprove a hypothesis.

Anecdotal reports are not usually falsifiable, as they are not collected in a fashion that may be repeated. A falsifiable observation must, by definition, be repeatable. Individual reports based on observed phenomena, are often subjective, and rarely controlled. Anecdotes that are emotionally charged, unusual and interesting are often given greater weight than would seem plausible.

Box 3.2. Success: anecdote and cervical cancer

The statement 'Nuns don't get cervical cancer' has often been quoted, and perhaps may not even be a correct quote of the Italian paper it is ascribed to. Rigoni-Stern is credited with saying this in 1842. Many research articles on the epidemiology of cervical cancer mention the work of this surgeon in Padua working in the mid-nineteenth century, who appears to have had an amateur interest in epidemiology.

Drife (1984) stated about cervical cancer that '… it is now well documented that the disease is rare in nuns and common in prostitutes … a connection between intercourse and cervical cancer was apparently first suggested in 1842.'

Is this what was reported? Rigoni-Stern published his ideas in a regional medical journal. It was impossible for Rigoni-Stern to make any comments on the incidence of deaths from cervical cancer. He did find four deaths from cancer of the womb among 1288 deaths in nuns, where it has been calculated later that six would have been expected (Skrabanek, 1988). Rigoni-Stern did not draw conclusions from these data that have been ascribed to him subsequently. He limited his observations on cancer to noting that the ratio of deaths from breast cancer to deaths from cancer of the womb was far greater in nuns (and single women) than in other women. This observation, of an excess of breast cancer in nuns, had already been made almost 150 years earlier by Ramazzini in 1713.

How such misquotation comes about is difficult to understand. Although the paper is written in Italian, there is no lack of clarity about his findings. These anecdotes were clues to the possible cause of cervical cancer, but they must be interpreted with care.

Box 3.3. Anecdote

A friend is talking about a party they went to at the weekend for a great-uncle who just turned 92: 'He's such a great character, always laughing. Do you know he still smokes 50 cigarettes a day? It may be a bad habit, but he's still alive – and they say tobacco is bad for us! If it was that bad he would have died by now.'

This is always a difficult concept to explain. The instance above is a single story about a lucky man – his risk of dying prematurely is greatly increased by smoking, and many of his peers in the same situation will have died. It is just that he has been lucky and has not succumbed to the probability of death. In science we call this an anecdote. Anecdotes can be useful for offering observations that generate research questions, but they cannot provide any useful evidence for a scientist.

The placebo effect is a well-known phenomenon where a patient's expectations may affect the outcome. Any observations, based on a clinician's or a patient's views, may be based on the effects of the placebo. Other forms of rigour in collecting data are absent from anecdote. For example, it is often difficult to collect information in an objective sense, on information to do with illegal recreational drug use, or sexual habits. Anecdote on these subjects may be biased.

Courts of law differ to science in their interpretation of evidence

A court of law examines the testimony of witnesses through checking for credibility, corroboration and cross-examination. However, replication is not seen as an essential method for testing legal evidence. These methods would not be used in a scientific investigation.

Courts are often involved in determining the efficacy of evidence for medicine and science. A useful test, used in medical court cases in the UK, is the Bolam test: a court of law will accept a clinician's witness statement where a majority, over 50%, of clinicians would agree with your decision.

Strengths and weaknesses of the design

Anecdote, even one structured by case series, is a quick and easy way to begin the development of a hypothesis. It has a role in new disease surveillance and provides research with leads. It may provide the first recognition of previously unobserved conditions, and new insights, particularly into emerging and new diseases to medical science. Anecdote may also generate new avenues for determinants of disease that have not been pursued by epidemiology in the past.

The main weakness is that anecdote does not provide a formalized and objective method for generating and testing new hypotheses. We have argued that it may be used as an initial observation in the scientific method of working, but it has no scientific basis for testing hypotheses. As such, it is seriously affected by observer bias and should not be used for inference of the cause of a disease.

Summary

Anecdote has a role in epidemiology and clinical sciences. It has managed to identify the emergence of new diseases, for example HIV/AIDS. It has also caused some damaging science and interpretation of science to occur. All anecdotes should be treated with caution.

Self-test questions

Q 3.2.1: Explain why anecdote cannot be tested by science.

Q 3.2.2: Give an example of anecdote that was used in epidemiology.

Q 3.2.3: True or false? Anecdote is never falsifiable.

3.3   Case Report, Case Series

- Pre-requisite sections: 1.1, 2.1, 3.2.
- Learning outcome: By the end of the section you should be able to identify the uses and abuses of reporting individual patient stories.

We examine here case reports and series separately to anecdotes *per se*, as they are an established part of the medical and surgical method of working. Many journals allow medical professionals to publish written reports. This allows a level of peer review, not seen in other forms of anecdote.

As a background, case reports were used in social geography, developed by Pierre Guillaume Frédéric le Play, suggesting society cannot be studied as a single unit but we must focus on some element of society using multiple data sources. Le Play did this with families in a vast array of circumstances with an interest in their budgets.

Hamel described how the relative size of the sample does not magically transform these cases into a macroscopic work, avoiding the limitations of case study methodology. By establishing parameters, as applied in all good research, even a single case could be considered acceptable, provided it met the established objective. He was proposing the transformation from the local to the global for explanation.

Robert Park also worked like this in Chicago with a focus on poverty and deviance. His aim was to see beyond documents to see and talk with people in the field. 'Go and sit in the lounges of luxury hotels and on the doorsteps of the flophouses; sit on the Gold Coast settees and on the slum shakedowns; sit in the Orchestra Hall and in the Star and Garter Burlesque. In short go and get the seat of your pants dirty in real research' (Park, 1927).

There are methodological concerns when using cases of disease. The first question is which method to use i.e. an inductive or deductive method? Am I looking to gain insight into laws or establish cause through the elements of the case I already know? How generalizable is the case? A good question to ask at this stage is 'am I clear as to why this particular case was chosen?'. In investigating the phenomenon how do we tease out the elements we are interested in as integrated contexts are common? The context is important for identifying whether a phenomenon is isolated or replicated in other areas. The question that is always asked is 'do I need another case?'.

The case report is an important stage in recognizing disease

A case report is an empirical inquiry that investigates a contemporary phenomenon within its context; however it occurs often when the boundary between the context and phenomenon is not clear. Case series lack formal hypotheses and a formal study design defining the sampling criteria and methods. Other aspects such as a method for data collection, and analyses are also not defined beforehand.

A case series is rarely the best design to answer a research question, especially when describing clinical experience with an intervention, as there are so many things that need to be controlled for. Even when we think that an intervention is the best clinical or practical response to an event, drawing conclusions from a case series has limitations and allows few generalizable conclusions to be drawn. A case series, even when compared to a control group, cannot answer many questions about appropriateness, effectiveness and adverse events.

In the early stages of a response to a major event or disease outbreak, case series can provide useful and preliminary information for clinicians and policy makers. Uses for case studies include educating, illustrating, exploring, describing, explaining and synthesizing.

Imagine a situation where you are confronted with disease many thousands of years ago. We now take for granted that we are now able to distinguish different diseases; this is the first step towards recognizing that the disease may be cured. In order to do this, practitioners of western medicine have reported on individuals and the diseases, symptoms and signs they demonstrate.

A case report is done by a clinician when they want to describe a novel occurrence of a disease in an individual. The report will contain details of the symptoms and signs of the disease, possible diagnosis and differential diagnoses, and any treatment and prognosis used or available. The reason for a case report may be to report a new or unusual presentation of an already recognized disease. An unusual approach to treatment, either successfully or unsuccessfully, should also be reported to help future patients. Case reports may also point towards the reason a disease develops, or a situation where the disease occurs in combination with another condition. Box 3.4 summarizes a case report that impacted on neurological science, identifying that damage to certain parts of the brain may change behaviour of the individual.

A case report would be classified as a piece of anecdotal evidence and there are questions over rigour and selection. The report, being on an individual, may be an extreme version of that condition and this novelty may propel it into the literature. However, case reports have a role in maintaining vigilance for new and emerging diseases.

The case series is a more systematic collection of reports

A clinician may study a group of cases, extending the original case report to many individuals, known as a case or clinical series. In practical terms, a common approach to a case series is for the clinician to record observations on consecutive patients that fit the criteria for the series. This will regress the series towards the mean of the true underlying group, and hence make it less based on a sensational single case. It is also feasible for a report to be based on non-consecutive patients, but this returns to the subjective nature of choosing the most interesting cases rather than reporting on the true situation.

The case series may report on a new or emerging disease, as occurred in the series of patients with what was subsequently named AIDS. The series may show a common feature in an exposure that may be an underlying cause of the disease, or it may be a surprising reaction to a treatment that clinicians should be made aware of. As with all methods involving cases alone, the epidemiologist must be cautious about inferring causal mechanisms. The selection of cases, the lack of controls and the potential lack of repeatability make this method less useful than other more systematic methods.

Box 3.4. An example of a case report

Phineas Gage, born in the United States of America in 1823, survived an explosion whilst helping to build a railroad. A large iron bar was forced through his brain, destroying much of his left frontal lobe. Gage amazingly survived this, but suffered from personality changes. The observations and reports of Gage's injuries influenced thinking of physiology, particularly discussion about the brain. This single case, exceptional in the extreme, is still cited in psychology teaching.

However, case series may provide useful directions and insights that otherwise may not have been seen.

Some examples of bad science have led to controversial incidents for public health. The consecutive case series of developmental disorders in children reported by Andrew Wakefield, which was linked in the media to childhood vaccinations, led to a loss of public confidence in immunization strategies, and has led to outbreaks of some infectious diseases.

A group of cases may be named a 'cluster'

A cluster of something is where two or more events occur. This may be at the same time, or the same place or within some other entity. Clusters of disease are important for public health; they sometimes become politically important events. A disease cluster exists where there is a greater than expected number of disease cases in the same place within a reasonably short time frame, or within the same occupation.

The recognition of a large number of cases of haematological malignancies near to the Sellafield nuclear reprocessing plant in England led to political pressure being put on the government. The government-funded Black enquiry led to the setting up in 1987 of the Small-Area Health Statistics Unit (SAHSU), charged with examining risk of disease in relation to environmental factors. The cluster continued to be investigated by other agencies, including the government organization Committee on Medical Aspects of Radiation in the Environment (COMARE) that reported in 2003.

Aldrich and Sinks (2002) suggested a hierarchical classification system for clusters, with the top and most frequent level being a 'perceived' cluster. This describes the initial report of an aggregation of cases, no matter the source. Historically, most perceived clusters have not been identified through routine surveillance of disease in a community, but rather through public and clinician anxiety, media reports and, more recently, the promise of litigation. A subset of clusters may be deemed 'observed' and therefore worthy of further investigation. A subset of observed clusters may be classified as 'etiologic' clusters, where the aggregation of cases is suggestive of a causal factor.

The Texas sharpshooter fallacy

An infamous story gives this fallacy its name. In Texas, many years ago, a gunman was shooting his revolver at a wall. Once he had fired all six shots, he went to the wall and got out a piece of chalk. Then he drew a target around the bullet holes. This sharpshooter was identifying the target after having made the shots.

Box 3.5 shows how this is an inappropriate way to identify clusters. The identification of clusters may be open to a fallacy where the person identifying the cluster is led there through drawing their own boundaries. When a person identifies what they think may be a cluster, then that person may make the cluster look more impressive through designing the boundaries to fit the data. For example, it may be possible that through hunting through records you may find other disease cases in the vicinity years earlier. Then the temporal boundaries of the cluster would be expanded to include the earlier time frame. This fallacy illustrates why clusters must be carefully explored and inference can only be exploratory.

> **Box 3.5. Texas sharpshooter fallacy**
>
> Imagine a similar scenario to the sharpshooter above where you are throwing snowballs at a wall. You throw three, and they each leave a white mark.
>
> You couldn't say you'd hit the target, because there wasn't one. If you drew a target around the three marks, you still couldn't say you'd hit the target as the snowballs were thrown first. This is what happens sometimes with investigations into clusters of disease – a number of cases of a disease are observed, sometimes as few as two, and someone draws a target around these events and says that it is significant. This is known as the 'Texas sharpshooter fallacy'.

Does a cluster suggest an infectious aetiology?

Some epidemiologists conclude that clusters of disease, with indicators of interpersonal contact, suggest that infectious disease underlies the aetiology of the disease. The difficulties involved in identifying clusters of chronic disease have been discussed extensively. Rothman (1990), a critic of cluster investigation, pointed out that clusters have been useful in identifying previously unknown disease entities and their cause. He also commented that these were rare situations or new diseases, and formal investigation of such striking clusters was unnecessary.

One way to understand that cluster investigation may elucidate the aetiology of a disease is to recognize that we are trying to establish whether a causal component clusters, which places a further restriction on the utility of a cluster to provide aetiologic insight.

Inference that infectious disease might have been involved in a cluster is often based on unusual community characteristics, examination of community patterns of illness, and population change. With no comparison group available, we are not able to assess the likelihood that patterns were unusual. Furthermore, the true link between community characteristics and infectious disease is based on supposition; this would benefit from assessment of the relations of infectious disease load, biologic effective dose, and immunity to community characteristics such as population increase.

It is clear that a single cancer cluster offers little knowledge about the cause of a disease. Clusters will remain an important public health issue and may provide evidence for the generation of new hypotheses. However, diversion of limited resources into detailed cluster investigations may not be warranted, particularly since there are a large number of reported clusters yet to be explained.

Summary

The case report has an important role to play in the development of western clinical practice. The peer-review process allows these reports to have a level of rigour above anecdote. Multiple case reports can be made simultaneously, and this produces a case series. There have been situations where a case series has been interpreted as having meaning for the causes, or aetiology, of a disease. These inferences must be treated with caution by scientists, despite the media not understanding the nuance required.

Some case series are interesting enough to be considered as a disease cluster. Disease clusters have also been interpreted to mean that the disease has an infectious aetiology. One observational study rarely provides enough good evidence to recommend changes to clinical practice or to health policy decision making. For certain questions, observational studies provide the only evidence. Recommendations from observational studies are always stronger when supported by other evidence.

Self-test questions

Q 3.3.1: In a case series:
A Incidence may be directly calculated
B Rare diseases can be investigated
C The odds ratio may be calculated

Q 3.3.2: A disease cluster tells you:
A That the disease is caused by an infection
B That the disease is caused by a point source
C Those lawyers are interested

Q 3.3.3: A group of residents notice that there are three cases of childhood lymphoma in one street. This may be due to:
A Chance
B Texas sharpshooter fallacy
C An infectious aetiology

3.4   Cross-Sectional Survey

- Pre-requisite sections: 1.1, 2.1, 3.1.
- Learning outcome: By the end of the section you should be able to describe the cross-sectional survey design and its limitations.

Box 3.6 uses a metaphor to explain the meaning of a cross-sectional designed study. The tomato in the metaphor could represent the entire population of people we are interested in examining for disease. Any population also exists over a period of time,

---

Box 3.6. Cross-sectional study metaphor

A cross-sectional study design can be illustrated using a tomato as a metaphor.

Start by imagining you have never seen a tomato before. How would you find out what it was like? You could look from the outside and describe its shape, size and colour, but this misses much of the detail of the fruit. Someone who dropped a tomato once tells you that the inside of the fruit contains some seeds, but this is just a single report – an anecdote. It is not evidence. It does however give clues to what you may wish to discover. Imagine now using a knife to cut through the tomato. This is the cross-section, and reveals details inside the fruit that were not observable before.

---

and in the metaphor the three-dimensional nature of the fruit allows us to express this. If we wished to examine the population at one specific time, then using a knife to slice through the tomato exposes the situation in the population at that point in time. The exposed part of the tomato represents the population we can examine using the cross-sectional survey.

Anatomy of the cross-sectional survey design

The cross-sectional survey records the number of people with a characteristic of interest at the moment in time of the survey. The aim is to record information at the same time, or within a short time frame, on a series of people. It is a common market research tool. Surveys of people in shopping malls asking you about your opinion on a product or a political party are cross-sectional surveys. In epidemiology the characteristic is often the occurrence of a disease such as asthma, or a risk factor such as smoking tobacco.

In practical terms, a researcher will choose a pre-defined population to sample from. Then at a specified time, the sample will be surveyed for the information that is required. For example you may wish to find out the number of people with asthma in a GP population. You will determine the time point for the survey and the method for observing the number of people with and without asthma, such as querying the computerized medical records.

Disease prevalence is measured

The cross-sectional survey is an observational study design: the scientist does not control the exposure or outcomes of those in the survey. The scientist counts the number of people with and without a disease or risk factor. Knowing the number of cases and the number of people without the disease gives the disease prevalence or point-prevalence at that moment in time. The prevalence is usually given as a proportion or number per population.

Prevalence studies, such as reported in Box 3.7, are used to plan public health services and to manage treatment at a population level.

New cases for most diseases will not be counted this way. The short time frames for the survey will not allow many, or any, new cases to appear. Returning to our example, were you interested in the incidence of asthma in this practice, you would

---

Box 3.7. Cervical cancer and cross-sectional surveys

A large European collaborative study collecting data from France, Spain and Italy known as EUROPREVAL (Verdecchia *et al.*, 2002) measured the total prevalence, per 100,000 people of cervical cancer. They found that the disease was found in 109 per 100,000 women in France, higher in Italy at 106, and lower in Spain at 87.

These results tell the health services how many people are in an area with a disease, informing resource planning.

---

have to look back in time for a sufficient period to accrue incident cases of asthma. The practice population during this time would also inevitably have lost people, both with and without asthma, through migration and death, and accrued people who should not be counted.

Prevalence studies may be used for causation

The prevalence study, using a cross-sectional survey design, may be used to explore the causes of disease. The researcher can identify people with and without a disease, and then on these people may collect data on the levels of exposure to putative risk factors. The association between disease prevalence and risk factors can be calculated.

The main issue with using prevalence studies for causation is that the point at which the study is conducted does not reflect the point in time of the development of the disease. There are multiple reasons why the prevalence of disease may differ to the incidence of disease, in ways associated with the risk factor. The rate of cure or recovery may be associated with the factor or death or migration from the population. It is not straightforward to disentangle these competing effects on the prevalence of the disease, to allow the researcher to clearly see the incidence.

A series of cross-sectional surveys becomes longitudinal

Cross-sectional designs can be contrasted with longitudinal studies. A cross-sectional study is one that takes place at a single point in time. A longitudinal study is one that takes place over time; we have at least two, and often many, measurements in a longitudinal design. This sort of design is able to look at time trends, and can correlate events in time with disease incidence. Were a researcher to conduct multiple cross-sectional surveys, this could be considered a form of longitudinal design, although it is more common for the same people to be tracked over time.

The census is a cross-sectional survey

A national census, as is conducted in many countries, is a way for the government to decide how many people reside in different parts of their territory. Indeed the word statistics is derived from the word state, where the government counted the people to inform them of their resources and burdens. The age and sex profile of these people, and often more detailed information on demographic, socio-economic and occupational profiles, are collected. The census is a cross-sectional survey, in that it generally collects the data for a specific time point, often on one day.

Censuses are classified as routine data. Routine data is data that is collected, but not necessarily for the purposes of epidemiology. The routinely collected data may be used by epidemiologists, and this is often an attractive way to use data for low cost to the funding body. The main problem with using such routine data is that the scientist must often compromise; routine data does not often match the exact specifications that would have been developed for a study.

Strengths and weaknesses of the design

The biggest strength of the cross-sectional survey design is that it is usually the cheapest way to ascertain the numbers of people with a disease, or the risk factors for a disease. This is because there is no need to wait for disease to happen, or to hunt for specific numbers of people with and without a disease. A snapshot of the situation at that point is taken, making the design fairly rapid for collecting data.

The design allows the researcher to estimate the prevalence of a disease, which is useful for planning healthcare resources. The design does not lend itself naturally to elucidation of causality; whilst exploratory research may be useful, it should be interpreted with caution. The survey only represents that point in time, and does not take into account temporal changes in the prevalence. The design may be prone to influences on the sample, such as survival, cure, death or migration. These influences mean that using this design for studies of causality is fraught with difficulties.

Summary

A cross-sectional survey examines disease or exposures at a particular point in time. This is in contrast to other study designs, such as longitudinal studies that look at the variables of interest more than once in a time period. A cross-sectional survey can calculate prevalence, not incidence. There are a number of disadvantages of this type of design, in particular the inability to measure incidence and disentangle possible cause from effect.

Self-test questions

Q 3.4.1: Can a cross-sectional survey measure incidence or prevalence?

Q 3.4.2: Prevalence is changed by which (one or more) of the following:
A Deaths
B Cure
C Out-migration
D In-migration

Q 3.4.3: Taking regular exercise has been shown to cut dementia risk in women aged 50 and over. A GP practice covering over 10,000 patients identified 2,500 women aged 50 and over on their lists and posted them an exercise survey. Of the 1500 who returned the survey 850 reported taking part in regular exercise. What was the estimated prevalence of regular exercise in women aged 50 and over?
A 34%
B 0.6%
C 57%
D 25%

Q 3.4.4: Disease X is incurable. It is known that the incidence of disease X has been constant during the past 30 years. Researchers have determined that the prevalence of disease X is higher today than it was 15 years ago. Select the answer that best explains this observation:

A Patients with disease X had a shorter life span 15 years ago compared to today
B Patients with disease X lived longer 15 years ago compared to today
C The risk of getting disease X has decreased during the past 15 years

3.5   Disease Registers and the Ecological Study

- Pre-requisite sections: 1.1, 1.5, 2.1, 3.1.
- Learning outcome: By the end of the section you should be able to describe the ecological study design and its drawbacks.

Last's definition of epidemiology describes two key actions of an epidemiologist: recording the distribution and discovering the determinants of disease. The first of these requires knowledge of where the disease occurs and in whom. The cross-sectional survey is a tool that allows us to estimate the prevalence of disease, but a more useful measure of disease is incidence. Incidence describes the number of new cases of a disease, which removes the effects of cure, death and migration that the estimate of prevalence is prone to.

Incidence is most commonly measured using the disease register. This tool allows us to keep a record of the occurrence of new diseases. There is a large array of disease registers around the world that encompass a wide variety of diseases. The registers have some key common characteristics but also differ in many aspects including their size, quality, purpose, topic, cost and funding source. Irrespective of their differences, registers can be used for epidemiological research and health needs assessment, as a tool to improve care, and to improve service quality.

There is sometimes confusion over the terms 'register' and 'registry'. The disease register is the database that records the information about the new cases. The registry is where the register is located, the buildings, the personnel, the management, all of the infrastructure required to run the register.

The anatomy of the disease register

Disease registers are set up to record details about each new case of a disease, known as an incident case. These records allow us to estimate the rate of incidence of a disease. Registers operate in a pre-specified population over a defined time period, by counting the number of new cases. The number of new cases forms the numerator in the calculation of incidence, the top part of the equation. This is divided by some measure of the underlying population, known as the denominator, giving the rate of incidence for that disease.

An important feature of registers is when a register is defined as 'population-based'. Under these circumstances the register aims to count all new cases of that disease of interest within a specified population.

Along with the pre-defined place and time, the clinical and demographic definitions of a case are important. The case definition may have exclusions, as with other study designs. A further complexity that must be seriously considered is the changing practice of identification and diagnosis over the time frame that the register collects cases. Medical sciences have advanced dramatically over past decades and diagnostic techniques have changed and improved.

For example, the development of magnetic resonance imaging (MRI) in the 1970s, and its widespread use in developed-world hospitals since then, has changed the ability of the clinician to visualize soft tissue within the brain. Many brain and nerve disorders, such as multiple sclerosis (MS), have been detected earlier and with greater certainty than before the use of this technology. A register of MS over this period will have different degrees of identification of people with MS. The researchers must take this into account as you may find a dramatic increase in the number of people diagnosed with MS, which may not reflect a true increase in the incidence, but an improvement in the identification of new cases.

Allied with the changes to clinical diagnostic practice, are changes to coding systems over time. All diseases can be coded, and there are many systems in use. The World Health Organization's (WHO) International Classification of Diseases (ICD) has origins in the 1850s, with the first edition published in 1893. The WHO took over control of the classification with the sixth edition in 1948. The tenth version of the ICD was published in 1992 and continues to provide the international standard diagnostic classification for epidemiological and health management purposes. Many other systems are available, with classifications providing more detail and finer groupings for specific diseases, such as the cancer classification systems.

Registers identify cases from many different sources

The researcher designing a register must identify sources to ascertain cases; sources will depend on the local circumstances, the disease of interest and the finances. Some countries have diseases that, when identified by a clinician or laboratory, must be notified to an official organization by law. This information is used to monitor the disease, usually contagious and infectious diseases, and provides early warning of epidemics. The WHO introduced the International Health Regulations in 1969 requiring the reporting of three main diseases: cholera, yellow fever and plague. These reporting systems, which vary from country to country, may be used as a disease register.

Official reporting provides sources for a register in only a limited number of diseases. The epidemiologist needs other sources to recruit new cases of disease onto a register for most diseases. Clinicians provide an obvious place to recruit new cases of disease; they may be based in hospitals or the community. Many healthcare services have electronic database management systems that can be used to identify people with disease. For example, in the United Kingdom all episodes of a patient staying in hospital are recorded with information about the reasons for the stay and any other health related information, known as hospital episode statistics (HES).

Patients' support groups can provide an ideal source of cases for a register. Internet-based social networking has provided a more widely accessible source of data. Registers have used the media and newspaper advertising to recruit people, particularly for diseases or conditions where there are no obvious sources of cases.

Registers are used for many different purposes

The register study design has many different applications, such as

- Patient care, which improves when clinicians can review patients, their treatment and diagnosis, and recall them to clinic where necessary. Groups of patients may be monitored, for example those at high risk of developing further morbidity. Managers may monitor and plan for demand of services, communicating with patient groups and planning access.
- Public health relies on good data to monitor disease incidence, to plan intervention and to evaluate impact on health burden.
- Research, particularly into the causes and aetiology of disease, which is advanced when registers generate and test hypotheses of putative risk factors.

These diverse needs and applications of a register require a multidisciplinary team, stable funding, focused aims, comprehensive data collection systems and a design that relates well to function of the registry itself. Arrangements for access to the data, data security, accountability and reporting should be established before the registry starts to collect data as these will be important for the everyday running of a registry.

Issues of consent drive register design

In practice, informed patient consent is an important issue for registers. Where identifiable data are used, patients' consent to be included on the register usually needs to be sought, although, around the world, there are exceptions to this. For example, in England, consent is not required for the cancer registries to record details about each person diagnosed with cancer.

Any requirement for consent leads to the situation where consent may be withheld. There are good reasons for this, for example where there are mandates to report to life assurance companies, or when the distress caused by contacting every person who may have a disease outweighs the public good of completing this exercise.

It is difficult to operate a registry with fully anonymized data and although there are ways to link data we often need to use a unique identifying characteristic for each case. This can help to avoid double counting, establish cause and effect for a case over time, compare the register against other external sources of data and make linkages with, other unrelated, data sets possible in order to test research hypotheses. In this case 'anonymized', when used to describe information pertaining to an individual, means that the identity of that individual has been concealed or protected, whether by presenting such information in a statistical form or otherwise, such that it cannot be readily discovered or ascertained from that information.

Knowing how many we have missed uses ecological techniques

This brings us to one of the most difficult parts of running a population-based register. Knowing how many people we have missed in recruiting, known as ascertainment, is essential. However, as Donald Rumsfeld pointed out in 2002, there are known unknowns and this is one of those situations. We know that it is practically impossible to recruit every single person in a population with disease: there is no perfect recruitment method.

This has been a problem that the science of ecology has dealt with using statistical techniques known as capture-recapture. An ecologist knows that it is virtually impossible to count every animal or plant of interest within the study area. An ecologist visiting an area may use a trap to capture animals of interest, and each individual captured animal is labelled. Then they will release the animal back into the environment. The ecologist then allows sufficient time to pass so that all of the captured animals can return to their habitat. The ecologist will then return to the environment and attempt to capture a second sample using the same technique as before. Within the second sample there will be some animals that had been marked in the previous survey and these are known as recaptures. There are also some animals that have not been captured previously and may be marked.

The capture histories can be analysed statistically to estimate the size of the population without needing to capture the entire population. This same technique can be used to establish a disease register where the scientist cannot be certain that they will be able to capture all members of the disease population. Rather than using a trapping method for humans the epidemiologist can use lists of people with disease and compare the lists which an individual appears on. This is equivalent to capturing and marking the person. The lists will be the same sources that are used by the epidemiologist to recruit cases to the register.

When there are two sets of data on capturing people with the disease the Lincoln–Petersen method may be used. This assumes that the population under study is closed; individuals do not leave an area for example through immigration or through death. Individuals must also not be added to the area through being born or being newly diagnosed. This is obviously unrealistic for epidemiology, and these issues make this method less reliable than for ecologists.

With these assumptions in mind the proportion recaptured in the second sample should be the same as the proportion captured for the whole population. So in symbols:

$$\frac{r}{c_1} = \frac{c_2}{n}$$

where n is the estimate of total population size, c_1 the total number of people captured by the first list and marked on the first list, c_2 the total number of people captured on the second list, and r the number of people captured on the first list that were then recaptured on the second list. Through a simple rearrangement, the total population size n is

$$n = \frac{c_1 c_2}{r}$$

There are less-biased estimators and because in epidemiology we usually have more than two lists to compare it is more common to use log-linear modelling which allows more elaborate statistical models to be fitted to the data.

Incidence of disease is calculated for subgroups of the sample

One of the main outputs from a disease register is an estimate of the incidence of disease. An epidemiologist will often calculate incidence in a whole population and then will often wish to calculate incidence for subgroups of the population. For example, an atlas of disease may be compiled where incidence is calculated for smaller geographical areas and displayed on a map. This allows us to spot patterns in disease distribution and also for planners to assign resources.

The methods by which incidence is calculated vary depending upon the aims of the research. However the most commonly used for reporting incidence is number of new cases per unit of population per unit of time.

Causality is explored using the ecological study

There is a study design with a confusing name – the ecological study – which uses the data from a register and compares the incidence rates to some putative risk factor. In this study design the unit of observation is a subgroup of people rather than an individual person. This does not have anything to do with the science of ecology, and nothing to do with the use of capture-recapture techniques that were first developed by ecologists.

A simple ecological study is where the disease incidence in a series of regions is compared with some factor hypothesized as a cause of that disease. The comparison may be made graphically, or simply using some form of correlation or regression. For example, you may look at the association between smoking and lung cancer in different countries. A simple plot of the proportion of adults who smoke in a country against the incidence of lung cancer in that country may provide insights into the disease process.

The population subgroups may vary in their composition. They may be as large as countries, or specific age groups, or males and females. The ecological study does not have to use geographical comparisons; it may use any subgroup of a population. For example, the incidence of disease in different age groups within the population may provide important clues to the cause of disease. Many studies of disease within occupational groups may illustrate risk factors that have not been discovered previously and these fall within the ecological study design.

A successful ecological study was published in 1968 (see Box 3.8). Fraumeni and colleagues investigated the level of deaths from cervical cancer in nuns and compared them to the rest of the population (Fraumeni et al., 1969). The study showed a considerably higher proportion of deaths due to cancer of the cervix in the general population compared to nuns. The conclusion was that cancer of the cervix '… seemed related to coital factors'. This is a form of ecological analysis, combining all nuns to be the homogeneous group for risk factors for death from cervical cancer.

Assigning subgroup risk to an individual is the ecological fallacy

The question we must ask ourselves is 'what does this mean for a person living within a subgroup of the population?'. How does this relate to their probability of developing disease?

> **Box 3.8. Cervical cancer problem**
>
> An ecological study was published in 1968 looking at the issue of cervical cancer in Catholic nuns in the USA from 1900 to 1954 (Fraumeni *et al.*, 1969). The number of deaths from cervical cancer in the group of nuns was recorded and was found to be 11% of cancer deaths in 31,658 nuns. In the general population, 57% of cancer deaths in women arose in the cervix.
>
> The ecological assumption is that the rates of sexual activity are lower in nuns than the general population. The rates of death from cervical cancer are substantially different, and the authors concluded that this '… seemed related to coital factors'. This ecological study supported the original anecdotes with evidence.

When an ecological study compares a risk factor to the incidence of disease for that subgroup, it is putting all of the individuals into a single group. This is the 'ecological fallacy' which assumes all individual members of the subgroup exhibit characteristics of the subgroup at large. This is a form of stereotyping, in that we are guilty of the ecological fallacy when we infer characteristics about an individual from the characteristics of the group to which the individual belongs.

The ecological fallacy is a widely recognized bias inherent in the interpretation of data in an ecological study. Using a hypothetical example, let's imagine a study is done that shows that on average people living in city A were taller than those living in city B. This makes the assumption that a randomly selected individual from city A would be taller than a randomly selected individual from city B. Since the heights in the study were an average, it is possible that an individual from city A was in the bottom ten percent for heights and the one from city B was in the top ten percent.

For this reason, an ecological study is normally regarded as inferior to non-ecological designs such as cohort and case-control studies because it is susceptible to the ecological fallacy. Ecological studies can be easily confused with cohort studies, especially if different cohorts are located in different places. The difference is that in ecological studies there is no information available about the individual members of the populations compared, for example comparing several regions based on region-wide average air pollution and region-wide average prevalence of respiratory diseases, whereas in a cohort study the exposure and health is known for each individual.

Strengths and weaknesses of the design

Disease registers are widely used to describe the volume of new disease in a population. Many countries use them to monitor disease rates, such as the cancer registries in England. The main issue for any register, particularly one that attempts to be population based, is to understand the level of ascertainment of cases. The researchers must understand the local circumstances to most effectively recruit the highest proportion of cases into the register. If a register misses recruiting people, either equally across all members of the population, or worse still lower ascertainment in certain subgroups, such as certain ethnic groups, or in more deprived communities, an ecological study may be prone to bias. A register is also an expensive enterprise, particularly for rare diseases. This limits the number of diseases that have good registers, and the number of places in which this sort of epidemiological study can take place.

The data is sometimes collected without the permission of those in the study. For example, large cancer registers often do not seek consent from those registered with cancer. This makes the study less prone to participation, or selection, bias than other types of study such as the case-control study design.

The ecological study design, paradoxically, is seen as a fairly cheap and swift design. This is because many studies use existing data incidence, often publicly available or routinely collected, to compare to the risk factors of interest. The ecological study design uses disease data collected by disease registries, and the quality of the design is, in part, dependent upon the quality of the register. Our example of cervical cancer in nuns used data that was already collected, and the researchers were able to exploit this (see Box 3.8).

In spite of their weaknesses, ecological studies are useful because they can be carried out easily, quickly and inexpensively using data that are generally already available. If interesting and strong associations are observed, the results of ecological studies can provide the opportunity for later, more carefully designed studies (though more expensive and time consuming) to build on the initial observations.

The main bias inherent in the ecological study design is the ecological fallacy. This leads to the scientist assuming that population-level measures represent the individuals. Further aspects must also be considered, for example changes in coding practices, or improvements to diagnosis, particularly when comparing between registers, and over time.

Summary

The disease register is well placed for epidemiology to fulfil its first role, that is to record the distribution of disease. When defined as population based, the register must recruit as many people as it can from the defined study population. There are a number of obstacles to doing this, such as defining the coding systems, the diagnostic criteria and exclusions. Even when the epidemiologist has pursued all avenues for securing the most cases, it is not possible to know with certainty how many people have been missed. This is where capture-recapture techniques can be used.

The ecological study design is usually employed to compare the disease rates in a group of people to the average of a risk factor for that group. It is contrasted with designs where the risk factors and disease are measured for individuals such as cohort studies and case-control studies.

The ecological fallacy is an important drawback of this design. It leads to this design being used as a way to generate hypotheses, such as our cervical cancer example, rather than testing a hypothesis. However, despite these concerns the ecological study remains a popular design because it can use existing data for an efficient and cost-effective way to examine disease and risk factors.

Self-test questions

Q 3.5.1: A register collects:
A Incidence
B Relative risks
C Prevalence

Q 3.5.2: Describe the ecological fallacy

Q 3.5.3: You have general practitioner clinical data and hospital inpatient data for diabetes. Your general practitioner data finds 282 people with diabetes, your hospital data finds 209 cases. When the cases were compared it was found that 181 cases were recorded on both lists. How many people do you think have diabetes?

Q 3.5.4: What are the assumptions built into the answer for Q 3.5.3?

3.6 Case-Control Study

- Pre-requisite sections: 1.1, 1.5, 2.1, 3.1.
- Learning outcome: By the end of the section you should be able to describe a case-control study so that you should be able to identify whether a study has a case-control design.

The case-control study is a design that is straightforward for clinicians to understand. Box 3.9 discusses the design, describing how the case-control study is designed to discover the causes, or risk factors, for a disease.

Box 3.9. A clinician's approach

Imagine you are a busy clinician in a hospital clinic and you have just seen a patient with a rare form of diabetes. This has set you thinking: do we know what causes this disease? You decide to consult a textbook, and find that the causes of the disease have not been investigated. In this situation, how would you design a study?

As a clinician, you could recruit all of the people with this rare form of diabetes from your clinic. In medical parlance, these are known as the 'cases', and this would generate a list of people with the disease, known as a 'consecutive case series'. This may be useful, but you would also need to have an idea of what you thought may cause the disease. This is known as the exposure. You would need to come up with an exposure, or putative cause, which you wish to investigate. Let's say you suspect that the cause may be something personal to each patient, such as a component of their diets. You would need to take the dietary measurements of the individuals, which can be measured using a food-frequency questionnaire completed by each patient, or case. This would tell you the level of exposure in your group of cases. From this alone it wouldn't be possible to decide whether the dietary component causes this form of diabetes, you'd also need a comparison group. An individual chosen as a comparison is a 'control', and so this study design is called a 'case-control study'. To conduct the research you'd then compare the proportion of cases that are exposed to the proportion of controls.

A key characteristic of the case-control study design is that it is retrospective: the study takes place after the disease of interest has occurred (Fig. 3.1). It is an observational design because the researcher observes and measures and does not control the exposure or outcome of the people within the study. This study design is particularly useful for studying rare diseases. This is because in any one particular population it may take a great deal of time for sufficient people to be diagnosed with a rare disease to conduct a study. In the case-control study the researcher recruits all people they can find with a rare disease, and then recruits a group of controls who do not have the disease.

The study aims to represent the counterfactual population

An important criterion for any epidemiological study into causation is that we need a way to represent the counterfactual population. In other words, what would have happened to the identical population at the same time, but without the exposure present? Experimental study designs, such as the controlled trial, are able to manipulate two populations, the intervention and the control groups. The case-control study is observational, and so the control group must be chosen in such a way that it represents the counterfactual population. However, the two samples do not represent the population with and without exposure to the cause; they represent the groups with and without the outcome (see Fig. 3.1). This is subtly different to the counterfactual, with both exposed and non-exposed in the same group of cases and controls.

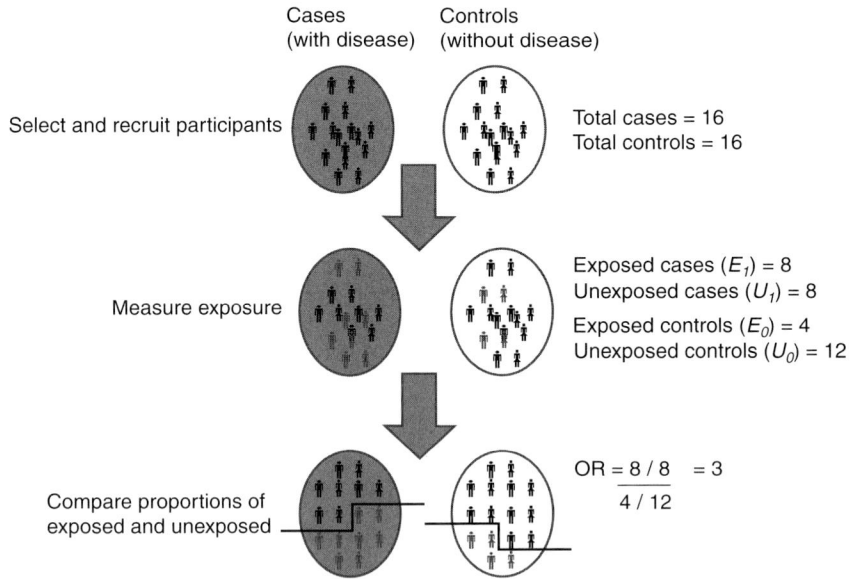

Fig. 3.1. The process of conducting a case-control study. People in grey are exposed to a putative risk factor.

Chapter 3

The study must fulfil the 'rare disease' assumption

The case-control design has an assumption that the disease under study is rare. An assumption of this kind means that the researcher must reassure themselves that the disease is rare, otherwise it makes the analysis, results and interpretation biased. The reason for this assumption is that the analysis of the study produces one measure of the relative risk, known as the odds ratio.

The rare disease assumption is a difficult concept because of the definition of rare. This is also referred to as an orphan disease. What constitutes rare? This is not a question that has an easy answer. As the prevalence of disease approaches zero the odds ratio also approaches the relative risk but, with any nonzero prevalence, which of course is required for the disease to be present in the population, the odds ratio deviates from the exact relative risk measured by the risk ratio.

Many rare diseases are due to the genetic makeup of the host, and for this reason often appear early in the life of the sufferer. In the United States of America, the Rare Disease Act of 2002 defined a rare disease by the prevalence in the population, as one that affects fewer than 200,000 persons in that country, which equates to approximately 1 in every 1500 people. In Japan, a rare disease is defined as affecting fewer than 50,000 people in Japan, equating to 1 in 2500 people. The European Union defines a rare disease as having a prevalence of less than 1 in 2000 people.

Case selection is important

The researcher must design a method to recruit cases into the study. This often proves straightforward with the close involvement of clinical colleagues. Cases may be recruited through clinic lists, or using a hospital clinical data management system. Where the disease under investigation is very rare, multiple centres may need to be involved to allow accrual of sufficient numbers of cases to fulfil the desired sample size. A particular type of case-control study, known as the incidence case-control study only includes new cases as they are diagnosed.

The researcher, under consultation with the literature and other clinical colleagues, should be aware of the need to exclude cases for certain reasons. For example, a case-control study into the causes of insulin-dependent diabetes should exclude all those people who have had their pancreas removed. Their reason for having diabetes is different to that for the majority of the population with diabetes.

Control selection is as important as case selection

Controls do not have the disease that we are investigating, making their identification and recruitment more problematic than for cases. Researchers often refer to controls as 'healthy controls' – which is a potentially misleading description. Any of the controls may have any other disease or condition, which does not preclude their involvement. The control group is designed to represent the 'base population'. This term was used by Wacholder and colleagues (1992a,b) to define the underlying population from which the cases were drawn. It is therefore important that the control group represents the same people who also may develop a disease of interest. If exclusions were applied to the case group then the same exclusions must be applied to the control group.

It is easy to underestimate the important part control selection plays in the study, particularly as the local medical professionals who are involved in the research are interested in the cases because they are the people they are treating. However, in the case-control study, the control group is as important as the case group.

There is no set ratio of the number of controls recruited compared to cases. It is commonplace for many studies to recruit a similar number of controls and cases. Power calculations demonstrate that a ratio of two controls per case gives better power. When a disease is rare, or cases difficult to find, or when cases die swiftly following diagnosis, the epidemiologist may have a higher ratio of controls to cases, which gives the study power without the difficulties in case recruitment.

Controls may be selected from many different sources, determined by local resources, the context in which the study has been performed, and the time and money available to the study:

1. Controls may be selected from locally, regionally or nationally available registers. These are generally known as population-based controls. For example, registers of births may be used to select a sample of controls that represent people living within the area. These registers are often very complete, and should not be affected by the disease under investigation. There may be ethical and legal issues with accessing such registers, and they will not contain immigrants into the area. Birth registers for studies of disease or exposure in children may be appropriate, however, the older a person becomes the less likely a birth register is to represent the base population. Other population-based registers include electoral rolls, tax registers and census records.
2. Another common sampling frame for controls is recruiting from the same neighbourhood as the cases. For example, on discovering where a case resides, the investigator visits the local neighbourhood and attempts to recruit a control from local housing, by knocking on the doors of neighbours. This will ensure that the controls are part of the geographically defined base population, and they may be representative of the socio-economic status of cases. The investigator must be aware that such controls may be associated with the cases, such as being genetically related.
3. Particularly popular in North America is the use of random digit telephone dialling techniques, where the investigator calls households using a random number generator. When an occupant answers the telephone an operator attempts to recruit the person as a control to the study. The success rate of this method is very low, as many people do not respond favourably to telephone marketing. This method also misses all people without a telephone, or people who are not available to answer the telephone at the time the call was made.
4. Clinicians may be tempted to use controls taken from hospital or clinical lists. For example a clinician may use a set of patients with a different disease to represent the base population. There are obvious difficulties with this approach; the potential controls are using clinical services for a reason, and may be affected by the exposure under study.
5. For some studies it may be appropriate to use close relatives, or friends, to represent the base population. Obviously exclusions on the basis of genetically related relatives must be made, if appropriate. The particular advantage of using this method is that friends and family are often very willing to participate in a study. A similar

approach may use non-genetically related spouses, husbands or wives, as they will have a similar environment but shouldn't have a similar genetic makeup.

Defining the exposure time frames with a pseudo-diagnosis

As we have discussed, the exposure to a putative risk factor must precede onset of the disease. In a case-control study, the investigator must define the time of diagnosis, so that the start and finishing times of exposure measurement can be made. As the controls represent the counterfactual population, the controls must also have a time defined as the start and finishing thresholds of exposure measurement. This is often referred to as the time of pseudo-diagnosis, and may be calculated in many different ways. The most obvious method is to calculate the exact age of a case at the time of diagnosis and use that exact age in the control, even though the actual calendar date is likely to be different between the cases and controls.

Matching is used to adjust for confounding

As with all observational studies in epidemiology, there is a threat of bias due to confounding in a case-control study. When a researcher is aware, or believes, that a particular variable is a confounder, the researcher may choose to match controls to cases on the basis of the confounding variable. For example, it may be suggested in the literature that age is a confounding variable for a particular disease. In a case-control study the researcher may match each control to a case on the basis of their age. Let's assume a researcher recruited a case who was 30 years of age, then the researcher may attempt to recruit a control who is also 30 years of age. During the analysis phase this matching must be taken into account using conditional analysis.

This approach has benefits for simplifying the method for calculating the time of pseudo-diagnosis for the controls. The exact age for each control is taken from the matching case. When matching is not done, the exact age then needs to be taken using some other method.

Amongst the drawbacks of this approach is the fact that the research is no longer able to look at the effect of the confounding variable on the disease risk. For example matching on age would mean that the researcher will not be able to examine the influence of age on disease risk. Further, it is necessary to identify correctly, and measure precisely, the confounding variable as it is not possible to change the design once the study has been conducted. Previous research may not have identified a true confounding variable, or may not know how precisely to measure the confounding variable.

Participation is a major threat to study results

Unlike laboratory studies, a case-control study, and indeed any health-related study, involves people and requires their voluntary participation. Participation, of the people you first select, is rarely 100%, and there is evidence that participation rates have been declining (Hartge, 1999). A particular problem for epidemiological research arises when participation is not randomly distributed across study groups. Unfortunately, whether or not an individual agrees to participate in a project is often associated with the health outcome and with the exposure(s) under investigation; invariably this leads to biased estimates of risk (Rothman, 1998). The assessment of the impact of differential participation requires the characteristics of those who do not take part to be compared with those who do. In most studies, however, information on non-participators is often sparse or non-existent. Indeed, in some designs, such as those that employ random digit dialling, investigators are not even able to identify non-participants (Wacholder *et al.*, 1992a,b).

There have been attempts to explore this form of selection bias that have relied mainly on re-approaching non-participants and asking a restricted number of questions (e.g. Holt *et al.*, 1991; Madigan *et al.*, 2000; Wrensch *et al.*, 2000). However, even when the identities of non-participants are known, practical and ethical considerations often prohibit the use of such methods. Other studies have used nationally available census data, such as the United Kingdom Childhood Cancer Study (UKCCS) which provided a valuable opportunity to investigate the potential impact of participation bias (UKCCS Investigators, 2000).

The issue of non-participation, and consequential bias that may be introduced, is critically important in case-control studies that rely on personal contact to assess environmental experiences and exposures. The UKCCS findings indicated that in such studies, the profiling of non-participants may be as important as that of participants. The involvement of parents in this study required active participation, as information was primarily collected through a face-to-face interview (UKCCS Investigators, 2000).

Motivation for controls to participate is not straightforward. As with all interview-based case-control studies, however, whilst the motivation of affected families to participate was strong, the motivation of those who were unaffected is less clear. Comparisons of census data for cases and first-choice controls provided results that were free from participation bias. The findings suggested that, on average, case families tended to live in areas that were more affluent than those of control families. In contrast, comparison with participating control families suggested that, on average, case families tended to live in areas that were less affluent than those of control families.

Cases and controls may differ due to participation effects

This observation is consistent with other reports suggesting that participants often belong to higher socio-economic groups than non-participants as measured by housing tenure, income, level of education and occupation (Holt *et al.*, 1991; Madigan *et al.*, 2000; Wrensch *et al.*, 2000). Measures of material deprivation are often closely associated with possible aetiological factors such as smoking, occupation and previous illness history. Indeed, in many epidemiological studies it is virtually impossible to identify potentially harmful exposures that are not – either directly or indirectly – related to measures of social class, deprivation or affluence. The challenge is to disentangle the artefactual consequences of participation bias from genuine aetiological factors. Some researchers have suggested using the variable most closely related to participation as a confounder to 'adjust' for participation.

For example, random digit dialling (Robison and Daigle, 1984) prohibits recruitment from homes without a telephone, those not at home when telephoned, and those who answer but who either refuse to answer any questions or deliberately lie about their family's eligibility. Differential participation is a potentially major source of bias in case-control studies that estimate risks on the basis of information reported from respondents alone. Studies that ignore this source of bias may produce misleading results.

Analysing the case-control study gives an odds ratio

As shown in Fig. 3.1, the proportion of cases and controls that are exposed is compared. In its simplest terms, the proportion of the cases exposed, divided by the proportion of controls exposed gives the odds ratio (OR):

$$OR = \frac{e_1/u_1}{e_0/u_0}$$

where e_1 and e_0 are the number of exposed cases and controls respectively, and u_1 and u_0 are the number of unexposed cases and controls respectively. See Fig. 3.1 for a worked example.

An odds ratio represents the relative risk, and for rare diseases is numerically nearly the same as a risk ratio. Using more modern techniques of regression models, logistic regression may be used to explore the association of the odds of the disease with exposure to single risk factors, and multiple risk factors simultaneously.

When an odds ratio of greater than one is found, the risk of the disease is associated with the risk factor. In other words, the proportion of cases exposed to the putative risk factor is greater than the proportion in controls. An odds ratio of less than one shows that the risk factor protects against the disease. An odds ratio of one shows that there is no association between the risk factor and the risk of disease.

Strengths and weaknesses of the design

The case-control study has a number of strengths; principally it is good for analytical epidemiology of rare diseases. In fact, this is an assumption of the measure of relative risk that it generates. It is fairly quick to conduct, as you do not have to wait for new cases to occur; you are looking retrospectively at existing cases. Many, many studies have used the case-control design because they are investigating a rare disease and this is often the only feasible approach.

Prime amongst the disadvantages is that the selection of controls is critical and this stage is prone to bias, both in terms of selection and in terms of participation. A practical problem is that it can be difficult to find a suitable control group. There are a number of possible sources of controls, but each has distinct advantages and disadvantages.

Epidemiology has also found the willingness to participate in health studies is reducing, and this has an impact on the quality of the study. Bias due to differential participation is an issue that is often ignored by researchers, but may have a serious impact on the results. Differences in recall between cases and controls, owing to the disease being present in the cases, may also lead to bias.

STROBE, which stands for STrengthening the Reporting of OBservational studies in Epidemiology, is an initiative of epidemiologists, methodologists, statisticians, researchers and journal editors collaborating in the conduct and dissemination of observational studies. STROBE has specific recommendations regarding quality reporting. When reporting the results, it requires the eligibility criteria, the sources and methods of case ascertainment and control selection to be given. Also to give a rationale for the choice of cases and controls is important, as it is for matched studies, giving the matching criteria and the number of controls per case. When describing the statistical methods it is important to explain how matching of cases and controls was addressed. In the results, it is important to report numbers in each exposure category, or summary measures of exposure.

Summary

A case-control study compares cases, those with the disease, to controls, those without the disease. These two groups are compared on the level of the exposure of interest. These data allow us to calculate an odds ratio, which is a measure of relative risk. Where an odds ratio of one is obtained, this shows there is no association between the risk of the disease and the exposure.

Box 3.10 gives an example of a case-control study that examined the causes of cervical cancer. This study, along with other exposures, examined the number of sexual partners in relation to the risk of cervical cancer. A positive association was found, suggesting the disease was caused by some sort of sexually transmitted exposure.

The study design in part relies on the disease being rare in the population, but the definition of rare is not explicit and the researcher must use their judgement when interpreting results from a case-control study. The cases are often recruited through the health systems in place. Controls, however, which should not have the disease of

---

Box 3.10. Cervical cancer problem

The investigation into the cause of cervical cancer gained pace in the 1980s. Researchers set up studies with greater validity than the incidence and prevalence studies, and in this way there have been many case-control studies of cervical cancer.

In the USA, between 1984 and 1987, 266 women with invasive squamous cell cervical cancer were given a sexual history questionnaire to complete (Slattery *et al.*, 1989). These were compared with 408 control women, who did not have cervical cancer. This study found that the odds ratio for cervical cancer in women with ten or more sexual partners was 8.99. This was statistically significant. The use of condoms had a protective effect for cervical cancer of 0.53.

The authors stated that 'These data support the hypothesis that cervical cancer is a sexually transmitted disease'.

---

interest, are often recruited from other sampling frames. These include lists of births, those registered to vote, or those on census records.

Overall, the case-control study has had many successful applications in epidemiology, and for the present it will continue to be used.

Self-test questions

Q 3.6.1: Controls in a case-control study of stomach cancer and vegetarianism are chosen because:
A They have stomach cancer
B They are all vegetarian
C None of them are vegetarian
D They do not have stomach cancer

Q 3.6.2: A case-control study found that the odds ratio for a foot ulcer was 0.84 for smokers compared to non-smokers. The outcome is:
A Smoking
B Case-control study
C Foot ulcer

Q 3.6.3: A case-control study found that the odds ratio for a foot ulcer was 0.84 for smokers compared to non-smokers. This means:
A Smoking causes foot ulcers
B The risk of a foot ulcer is increased for those who smoke
C The risk of a foot ulcer is lower for smokers

Q 3.6.4: Which of the following statements is correct for a case-control study?
A Ascertainment of cases is always prospective
B Cases and controls could be matched for the risk factors other than the exposure under investigation
C Risk ratio can be calculated directly
D The number of cases must equal the number of controls

Q 3.6.5: Which of the following is not a disadvantage of case-control studies?
A Selection bias especially if the study base is poorly defined
B Recall bias which can lead to differential measurement error
C Relevant only to common diseases

3.7 Cohort Study

- Pre-requisite sections: 1.1, 1.5, 2.1, 3.1.
- Learning outcome: By the end of the section you should be able to describe the cohort study design and identify that design in any given study.

A cohort is a group of people who share a common experience or condition. For example, people in a birth cohort share being born at a similar time or similar place, or both. Cohorts may be based on an occupation, for example a cohort of rubber workers working within the rubber industry. The cohort study uses the shared experience of the individuals to design a powerful epidemiological study. The study of a cohort is most often used to conduct research into the cause of a disease and the natural course of a disease. A cohort study is seen as an excellent study design, although it remains observational, but is closest of all observational designs to an experimental design. The cohort design does become an important alternative to experimental design when there are ethical or indeed operational constraints on experiments.

The anatomy of a cohort study

The cohort study begins with a definition and identification of the study population: the cohort. The scientifically most robust form of cohort will recruit members of the cohort and then follow them prospectively through time. However, the cohort could be recruited after the exposures and disease events have taken place. At the time point that is defined as the start of the cohort study, no person should have been diagnosed with the disease of interest; they should be free from the outcome (see Fig. 3.2).

The cohort is assessed for the exposure that is being investigated, which is often planned to be done as close to the start of the cohort study period as possible. This stops the disease we are interested in potentially affecting behaviour and the measure of the risk factor. In an example of a factory-based cohort, we may divide our factory workers into those that work on the shop floor exposed to a chemical that is giving concern and those that work in the offices who are not exposed to the chemical.

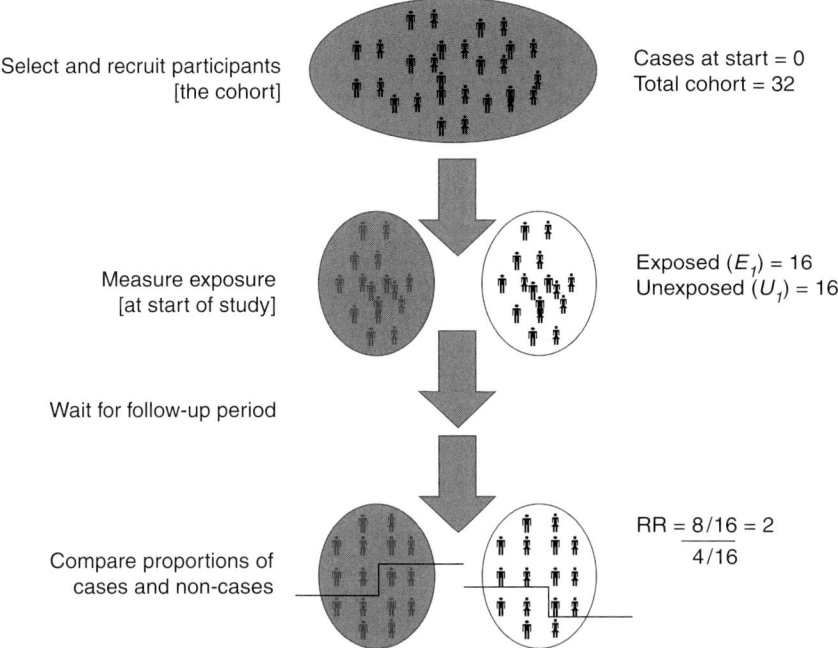

Select and recruit participants [the cohort]

Cases at start = 0
Total cohort = 32

Measure exposure [at start of study]

Exposed (E_1) = 16
Unexposed (U_1) = 16

Wait for follow-up period

Compare proportions of cases and non-cases

$$RR = \frac{8/16}{4/16} = 2$$

Fig. 3.2. The process of conducting a cohort study. People in grey are exposed to a putative risk factor.

The whole cohort is then followed through time, looking at whether the members of the cohort develop the outcome we are interested in. Cohort studies can be considered to be about the histories of individuals, and segments of their lives that are important for the outcome and exposure. The exact method for doing this will vary depending on the specific situation. The length of time that the cohort will be followed for will vary, again depending on how rare the disease is, and how many people were recruited to the initial cohort, but will often be a number of years. Returning to our factory example, the cohort may be straightforward to follow in the short term, as by definition you know you can observe them in their workplace. However, as time accrues, people leave their jobs, moving to new jobs, retiring or dying. This problem leads to 'loss-to-follow-up', and will be discussed later in this section.

Eventually, the researchers will have allowed sufficient time to recruit enough people with the disease. The risk of the outcome can then be compared between the exposed and unexposed groups. The comparison group may be the general population from which the cohort is drawn, or it may be another cohort of persons thought to have had little or no exposure to the substance under investigation, but otherwise similar. Alternatively, subgroups within the cohort may be compared with each other.

Choosing the members of the cohort is crucial

All cohort members must be at risk to develop the outcome or disease of interest. Similarly members must be free of the outcome at the start of follow-up. This does not mean that they must be healthy; they may indeed have other diseases and conditions. Cohort members are no longer at risk from the outcome if they die or if they develop the outcome. If the outcome occurs only once or confers lifelong immunity, then the participant is permanently excluded from the at-risk group. The cohort member may return to the at-risk group if the disease is curable and the disease does not confer lifelong immunity.

For the study to successfully recruit sufficient numbers of participants, the cohort must experience a range of exposures. Any cohort where the participants were either all ubiquitously exposed, or nobody was exposed will fail. There should be a balanced distribution of the exposure. Cohort members must also be available for testing the level of exposure to the putative risk factor, and for the people sampled to be followed through time to allow the study to identify the outcome in individuals. In this respect, the study has a longitudinal design.

There are many types of cohort

Epidemiologists have identified many types of cohort. The design and composition of each cohort will be based on a mixture of local circumstances, financial viability and the research question of interest. The cohort definition may be divided into some main types:

● A birth cohort is defined as the people born over a certain period of time, and usually within a specific location. There are many examples of these, for example in England there were cohorts that registered all of the people born in the whole of the country over a specific week, such as the 1970 birth cohort. These often form a cohort for studying a range of diseases and potential exposures.

- Workers in an industry may be recruited to an occupational cohort. These will be recruited because there is an interest in the health and safety of people working in a certain industry, or exposed to some putative risk factor.
- Some cohorts may be composed of people who were in a defined geographical place. A classic example is the survivors of the Nagasaki and Hiroshima atomic weapons. The members of this cohort all were exposed to the same exposure at the same time, and have been followed through time to provide important information about the consequences of ionizing radiation exposure.

Cohort studies may be prospective or retrospective

The design of the cohort can be prospective, with the participants followed through time. Or alternatively, there can be a 'records-only' historical cohort study. An example of this latter design might be an investigation of the mortality risk of children with birth defects by age at death, birth defect category and other possible contributing factors. We would firstly need access to all children born in a time period (for example 1980–2005) with reportable birth defects. These would all be included in the study cohort. A comparison population might be all births for that time period in another state. The deaths among the study cohort would need to be identified through linking cases to the death certificate files. Statistical methods could be used to calculate risk ratios (mortality risk) and adjust for selected infant and maternal risk factors.

A records-only prospective cohort study could be used to determine the demographic, environmental and medical factors that influence the weights of a newborn infant and the placenta and compare this ratio with other factors known to predispose to adult ill health. We would do this by beginning at a time period and collecting all data, for example by questionnaire from pregnant women and their partners, at a set point in gestation and again at a later stage of gestation. We could identify an association between a raised placental weight to birth weight ratio and hypertension in adulthood. We could also work out whether the gestational age is important when interpreting the placental weight to birth weight ratio, and assess how environmental factors are associated with changes in the placental weight to birth weight ratio.

A cross-sectional survey with routine data follow-up could be used to assess the impact of breastfeeding on the risk of obesity and risk of being overweight in children at the time of entry to school. Routine data at the time of school entry could be compared to responses to a questionnaire completed by parents regarding breastfeeding.

Historical records of exposure could be obtained with a special survey to measure disease outcome such as second-hand smoke (SHS) exposure and asthma health outcomes. SHS exposure during the previous 7 days could be measured using a personal nicotine badge and exposure during the previous 3 months estimated using hair nicotine and cotinine levels. Asthma severity and health status could be assessed using telephone interviews, and subsequent admission to hospital for asthma could be determined from health care utilization databases.

Risk ratio is the measure of association

The data collected from a cohort study can be expressed in a two by two table. For example, you would count the number of cohort members who had developed the disease and had been exposed. From this, we can calculate the relative risk. As shown in Fig. 3.2, the proportion of exposed cases and exposed non-cases is compared. In its simplest terms, the proportion of the exposed that are cases, divided by the proportion of unexposed that are cases gives the risk ratio (RR). To begin, we calculate the event rates, or rates of the outcome, in the exposed (EER) and unexposed (UER) groups as

$$EER = \frac{e_1}{e_0 + e_1}$$

and

$$UER = \frac{u_1}{u_0 + u_1}$$

where e_1 and e_0 are the number of cases and non-cases in the exposed group, and u_1 and u_0 are the number of cases and non-cases in the unexposed group respectively. The relative risk, estimated as the risk ratio (RR) is the ratio of these two event rates:

$$RR = \frac{EER}{UER}$$

Let's illustrate this with an example. Imagine a study where we wanted to ask whether gender has an effect on the likelihood of disability. Can you determine what the outcome is? In this example, disability is the outcome for this research question. What is the exposure? It is being male or female, and in this example we imagine that being male is the 'exposed' group. In our example, there were 409 males with a disability, 728 males without a disability, 193 females with a disability and 652 females without. Putting these together we discover that the risk of disease in males was *409/1137=0.36*, and in females was *193/845=0.23*. The overall risk ratio is *0.36/0.23=1.56*. In this example males have 1.56 times the risk of disability compared to females.

The risk ratio represents the relative risk. Similar to the odds ratio for the case-control study, modern techniques of regression models may be used to explore the association of the risk of the disease with exposure to single risk factors, and multiple risk factors simultaneously. When a risk ratio of greater than one is found, the risk of the disease is associated with the risk factor. In other words, the proportion of people exposed to the putative risk factor who are cases is greater than in the non-case group. A risk ratio of less than one shows that the risk factor protects against the disease. A risk ratio of one shows that there is no association between the risk factor and the risk of disease.

There are important and famous cohort studies

There are a number of important cohorts that have advanced public health:

1. The British Doctors' study was set up in the early 1950s to investigate smoking and its possible health consequences. It recruited 40,000 male clinical doctors from

Great Britain. All of these people, on recruitment, had not been diagnosed with a lung cancer. Their smoking habits were recorded and the cohort was followed until their death, and analysed by cause of death. The members of the cohort were followed up using further questionnaires in 1957, 1966, 1971, 1978, 1991 and finally in 2001.

2. The Framingham Heart Study was a US-based study into the causes of cardiovascular disease, with the residents of the town of Framingham, Massachusetts, forming the cohort. The cohort was recruited in 1948 with 5209 adult subjects. Before Framingham, very little was known about the causes and risk factors of cardiovascular disease. Much of the now-common knowledge concerning heart disease, such as diet, exercise and aspirin, is based on this cohort study.

3. There are a number of British birth cohorts, often remembered for the year in which the cohort was born. For example, the British Births Survey (BBS) 1970, now often referred to as the '1970 cohort'. Data were collected about the births and families of 17,000 babies born in England, Scotland, Wales and Northern Ireland in one week in April. The survey aimed to examine neonate morbidity, and relate this to social and biological characteristics of the child's mother. Recently, the Millennium Cohort Study (MCS) follows the lives of 19,000 children born in the UK around the time of the new millennium. Four surveys of the cohort have been completed: at age 9 months, 3, 5 and 7 years.

A case-control study may be nested in a cohort

A nested case-control study uses a defined cohort to select cases of a disease and the appropriate controls, those who have not been diagnosed with the disease. This approach usually offers the epidemiologist a well-defined base population from which to sample, which helps to reduce costs. The case-control study may also require information on aspects of the person's life that has been collected contemporaneously by the cohort study. This will reduce the potential for bias due to recall.

It may not be feasible to collect certain types of biological material, for example levels of folate in venous blood samples at the time of the birth of a child, retrospectively in a traditional case-control study. Embedding a case-control study in an existing cohort study may allow the examination of material already collected in a case-control design.

A major drawback of this form of design is when the cohort has low levels of participation. This often renders the cohort unrepresentative of the original base population. The resulting case-control study may be influenced by selection bias. When the epidemiologist is aware of this as a potential bias, non-random selection may allow the sample to return to more appropriate representation.

Household panel surveys are a sub-type of cohort study

A panel study draws representative samples of households and surveys them, following all individuals through time on a usually annual basis. Examples include the US Panel Study on Income Dynamics (since 1968), the German Socio-Economic Panel (since 1984), the British Household Panel Survey (since 1991), the Household,

Income and Labour Dynamics in Australia Survey (since 2001) and the European Community Household Panel (1994–2001). The reason to distinguish this from a regular cohort study is that the unit of interest is the household. Information of the members of the household is collected, and when the household moves residence, this is usually tracked and the household is surveyed in their new location.

Loss-to-follow-up weakens a cohort study

The cohort is followed over a time period and measured at least once, and usually periodically. The researchers on a cohort study will follow, or monitor, the members of the cohort. This may be done over a long period of time, such as the 50 years that the British Doctors' cohort was studied. During the follow-up period new questions may be asked that are relevant at different times. The level of the exposure may be measured again, to bring it up to date or to use newer methods to measure exposure status. Importantly the outcome that we are interested in, such as the disease, can be detected in the cohort.

Over the extended periods of time that the cohort is studied, the members of the cohort may be lost by the surveillance system, known as loss-to-follow-up. This is one of the most important sources of bias in a cohort study. People may be lost to follow up due to death, migration or a conscious decision to withdraw from the study. These may all have consequences for the quality of the data: losses of certain sections of a population, such as more affluent groups, will have an impact on the efficacy of the study to reflect the truth.

Strengths and weaknesses of the design

The cohort study design is perceived as the best observational study design. It is good at looking at diseases where rare exposures are suspected. It can be designed to look at multiple outcomes, unlike a case-control study which looks at only a single disease. The design cuts down on many forms of bias, such as recall bias. This is because, for example, the exposure information is collected in advance of any disease, and so there is no differential recall between those with and without disease. Also, unlike a case-control study, the incidence and risk of a disease is measured directly within the cohort. Unlike the case-control study, the measure of relative risk is a measure of risk, rather than odds.

The biggest drawback of a cohort study is that investigating a rare disease needs a very large cohort (Box 3.11). This problem leads these studies to be expensive and slow to accumulate sufficient disease cases. A further disadvantage is losing people as time moves on, which cuts down the size of the cohort and may lead to biased results.

STROBE (see Section 3.6) has specific recommendations regarding quality reporting. When reporting the results, it is important to give the eligibility criteria, and the sources and methods of selection of the participants. It is important to explain how any loss-to-follow-up was addressed. In the results, it is important to report and summarize follow-up time and report numbers of outcome events or summary measures over time.

> **Box 3.11. Unfeasible cohort**
>
> We've been looking at how epidemiology has helped prevent cervical cancer, and the question emerges, why was a cohort study of cervical cancer not done? It comes down to numbers.
>
> Eight per 100,000 people in England developed cervical cancer in 2007. Let's say for the sake of this demonstration we want to generate a sample size of 100 and get some results from the study in 5 years. If there are eight women with cervical cancer per 100,000 women per year, that will give 40 women over 5 years with 100,000 in the cohort. To reach the desired sample size of 100 would require 250,000 women in the cohort for the 5 years to produce 100 cases. In practical research terms these numbers aren't feasible so alternatives are considered instead. For example, a cohort to look at pre-cancerous lesions may be one alternative.

Summary

The cohort study is a powerful epidemiological design for examining putative risk factors for disease. A cohort, or more than one cohort, is identified by the epidemiologist. This may be based around a time or place of birth, a particular occupation or a geographically delimited area. The most robust designs identify the cohort before any of the outcomes have developed, or been diagnosed. This is an important aspect of the cohort, in that no member of the cohort when they enter the cohort must have the outcome of interest.

The exposures of interest are measured at the appropriate times, and the members of the cohort followed using surveillance systems. Then a measure of risk of the outcome in those exposed to the risk factor and those not exposed allows the calculation of the relative risk. This forms a measure of the strength of the change in risk between the two groups. More elaborate designs can be analysed using regression models.

The drawbacks of the design are, first and foremost, the cost of running a study for rare diseases. Many chronic and acute diseases will require many thousands of participants to generate sufficient power. This may be unfeasible for funders. The second drawback is the potential of loss-to-follow-up, where the participants are unable to be incorporated into the study, either for passive or active reasons. However, the cohort study remains the most powerful observational study design available to epidemiology.

Self-test questions

Q 3.7.1: Which of the following statements is correct for epidemiological studies with a cohort design?
A Cohort studies are most useful for investigating rare diseases
B Cohort studies are not subject to confounding biases
C Cohort studies can produce estimates of attributable risk
D Cohort studies require identification of all possible risk factors

Q 3.7.2: In a cohort study of Leeds school children, loss-to-follow-up
A Cannot occur for school children
B Happens to all children when they leave school
C Is not relevant
D May lead to bias that might affect the results

Q 3.7.3: Which one of these examples is a cohort study?
A A group of 200 men aged over 60 were randomly assigned to either attend a Tai Chi class once a week or not, the number of falls reported in each group was then compared
B Brain tumour patients and healthy controls were asked about their history of smoking in the previous 10 years
C Ten thousand pregnant women were recruited and information was collected on medication use throughout pregnancy until childbirth, the children were then monitored for 20 years to see how many went on to develop asthma
D The incidence of obesity in several European countries was compared to the average hours of TV watched per member of the population to see if countries with high levels of TV viewing had a higher level of obesity

Q 3.7.4: At the start of a birth cohort study looking at the association between breastfeeding and asthma
A All participants have asthma
B All participants will be twins
C None of the participants will be bottle fed
D Some participants will be breastfed

3.8   Randomized Controlled Trials

- Pre-requisite sections: 1.1, 1.5, 2.1, 3.1.
- Learning outcome: By the end of the section you should be able to describe the randomized controlled trial design and identify that design in any given study.

A 'randomized controlled trial', often abbreviated to RCT, is a scientific experiment used to determine how useful an intervention may be in the field or in the laboratory. The RCT may also sometimes be referred to as a 'randomized clinical trial' or 'controlled trial', where they probably refer to a similar design. An RCT can be used to test drugs, a service delivery model or any therapeutic product, not just for use in healthcare. An early example of an RCT was published in 1948 in a paper examining the use of streptomycin to treat pulmonary tuberculosis (Medical Research Council, 1948). One of the authors of that paper was Austin Bradford Hill, credited with developing the RCT design, who around the same time worked with Sir Richard Doll on the links between cigarette smoking and lung cancer.

The RCT is as close as you can get to an experimental study design within the constraints of human medical research. For this reason, it is seen as providing the most reliable form of evidence from a single study in epidemiology. This can be strengthened further by combining studies into a meta-analysis of studies.

Clinical trials are big business; they are required by the pharmaceutical industry and manufacturers of medical equipment for official approval and for healthcare organizations to justify spending money. The RCT design has become standardized and service-led, and is usually purchased through dedicated clinical trials units as an off-the-shelf product.

Returning to our overarching example (see Box 3.12), a preventative measure has been investigated for cervical cancer using an RCT. Prevention has been investigated using vaccines for human papillomavirus (HPV). The RCTs have shown that the vaccines are a successful way to prevent cervical lesions.

The study is designed to test an intervention

An intervention is used to alter or hinder an action or development in a given situation. An RCT is used to test how well an intervention works, with the scientist manipulating the intervention and hence the design is experimental. The intervention is determined by what the scientist wishes to test. Here are some examples:

- A scientist has developed a new drug to treat leukaemia. The epidemiologist tests how the new drug behaves in treating leukaemia. The drug is the intervention. The outcome of the trial will be the cure of leukaemia.
- A surgeon wishes to test a new surgical procedure to treat angina. The procedure is the intervention and the outcome successful treatment of angina.
- An epidemiologist wishes to test whether a new washing-up glove protects the user from developing eczema. The glove is the intervention and the outcome is prevention of the development of eczema.
- A psychologist wants to test whether cognitive behavioural therapy (CBT) will prevent addiction to video games. CBT is the intervention and the prevention of addiction is a successful outcome.

Anatomy of a randomized controlled trial

The first requirement for someone wishing to pursue an RCT, as with all epidemiology, is to define the study population (see Fig. 3.3). There are two main alternatives,

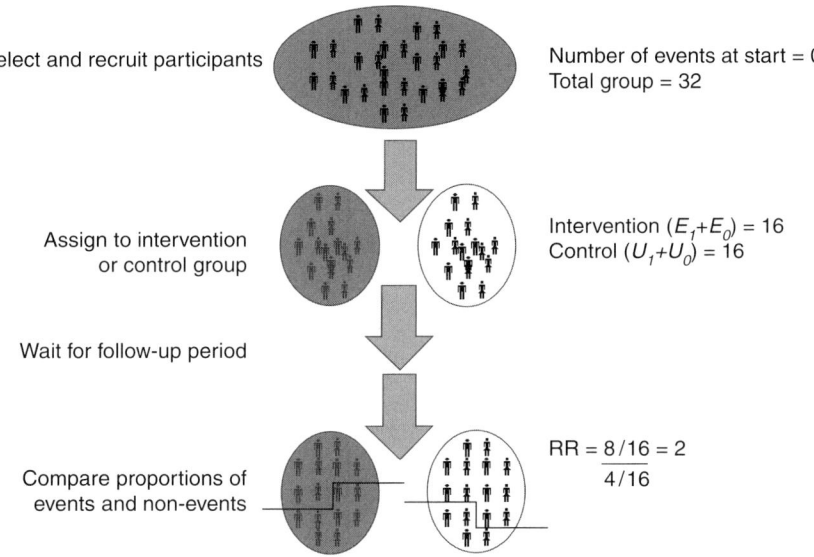

Select and recruit participants — Number of events at start = 0
Total group = 32

Assign to intervention or control group — Intervention $(E_1 + E_0)$ = 16
Control $(U_1 + U_0)$ = 16

Wait for follow-up period

Compare proportions of events and non-events — $RR = \dfrac{8/16}{4/16} = 2$

Fig. 3.3. The process of conducting a randomized controlled trial.

depending on whether the trial is assessing an intervention to prevent something, or whether the trial is designed to test an intervention where the outcome is to get rid of a disease, condition or exposure.

In the former case, all the study population will, at the start of the trial, be free from disease or condition of interest. We will refer to this as a prevention trial. For example, we may be testing the ability of aspirin to prevent a heart attack. In public health, this is known as primary prevention and at the start of the trial all participants have not had a heart attack.

In the second case, all of the study participants must have the condition that the intervention is designed to cure. This is a fairly standard requirement for the pharmaceutical industry in designing new therapeutic drugs and we will refer to this as a therapy trial.

Once the study population has been defined, recruitment of participants may take place. In a therapy trial designed to cure or remove a condition or disease, this is most often done through clinics, which often have an accessible source of people willing to be approached and recruited into trials.

Defining and identifying a sampling frame for a prevention trial may be more problematic. This is because the potential recruits are not being treated for a disease that you wish to eradicate; the potential recruits are often in the community and do not belong to a simple-to-access list.

An experiment uses a control group

The name of the study design describes some of its key points: let's begin with the word 'controlled'. In a simple RCT design there is one set of participants. They all have the same characteristics, or condition, that you are planning an intervention on. The study divides these participants into two groups, by a process covered in the next section.

You may choose to divide your study sample into two groups comprised of a 50:50 split. But the exact proportion in each group may differ depending on the local circumstances. One group is given the intervention under test; they would be referred to as the 'active', 'intervention' or 'treatment' group. The rest of the participants, not in the active group, are not given the real intervention. These form the control group. They may be given no intervention, or more commonly a placebo. A placebo mimics the active treatment but does not actually work in the same way as an intervention. Alternatively there may already be an intervention that works, and the RCT is designed to test which of the interventions is superior or non-inferior.

The control group allows a new intervention to be compared with existing interventions or with no intervention. Otherwise we don't know if any change in treated participants is due to the treatment rather than something else, such as a placebo effect.

Illustrating this with an example (see Box 3.13) there are three groups, two of which might be considered as controls. The first controls are the group that receive the standard treatment. The second control group is more interesting. These are given a treatment procedure that, to the patient, is experienced as real acupuncture, except the process is not correct to fulfil the requirements of traditional Chinese medicine.

The strength of the design is based on the term 'randomized'

The word 'randomized', in the name of the design, refers to the process or method by which the participants are assigned to a group. The person is assigned randomly to one of the groups, either intervention or control, without this being based on any other characteristic. Randomized in this sense refers to a probability of being assigned to a group. This must not be confused with random selection, also used in epidemiology, where a person has a probability of being selected for a study.

Each participant has a known chance, or probability, to be assigned to each group. The probability totals one for all groups that a person may be assigned to.

Box 3.13. An RCT to reduce osteoarthritic knee pain

A study by Foster and colleagues (2007) reported in the British Medical Journal used an RCT to examine acupuncture for reducing osteoarthritic knee pain. Three hundred and fifty-two patients with knee pain were recruited; all had an osteoarthritic knee and all received advice and exercise plans. These participants were randomized to no acupuncture, true acupuncture or sham acupuncture. Sham acupuncture is a form of placebo where they were attended to by an acupuncturist and needles were inserted in their skin. But they were not placed in the correct places according to the Chinese medical tradition. The change in pain scores at six months was measured. Throughout all of these groups, there was no significant difference in results.

A randomized process is used to avoid bias by the investigator. The randomization is one of the most critical parts of an RCT. It allows the study to avoid some forms of bias. For example, if a new drug was tested to cure a fatal disease, where none has existed before, an investigator, particularly a treating clinician, might put the most 'deserving' cases into the treatment group. They might choose younger people, or those with children, or those who were more seriously ill. This is human nature. However, this would also introduce a serious bias that would make the results uninformative. Randomization avoids this, by taking the act of assigning participants to groups out of human hands. A second benefit of the randomization process is that for other characteristics the groups are similar. They do not have to be identical, but sufficiently similar to avoid further bias.

If an RCT had two equally sized groups, an active treatment and a control group, then probability is 50% to be in each group. Returning to the acupuncture example (Box 3.13) the participants were randomized to one of three groups. The groups are designed to be similar in size, and so the probability of being assigned to each group is one third.

RCT designs can be categorized

There are many ways to design the randomization for an RCT:

- Parallel-group randomization, the most straightforward approach and that which has been described so far, is where each participant is randomly assigned to one of two groups. All participants in the intervention group receive the treatment, and all in the control group receive no intervention.
- Crossover randomization is where the participants begin in one of two groups, an intervention or control, and over time, each participant then changes, or crosses over, to the other group. There is often need to allow a period between the two arms of the trial, known as a 'wash-out' period. This allows the scientist to observe the effects of the intervention on all participants.
- Cluster randomization uses pre-existing groups of participants, such as schools, class groups within schools, towns or streets, which are randomly assigned to the intervention or control group. All members of a cluster receive the same intervention or placebo.
- Factorial randomization assigns participants to groups and each group is given a combination of intervention and placebo.

RCTs may also be classified into either explanatory or pragmatic. Explanatory RCTs test an intervention in a highly controlled research setting, with selected participants. It is not intended to test the intervention in a community setting. In contrast, pragmatic RCTs examine an intervention in the situation where the intervention will end up being used in everyday circumstances. These trials are designed to represent real-life situations.

A third method classifies the aim of the trial in comparing treatments: classification as superiority, non-inferiority or equivalence trials. In superiority trials, the intervention is hypothesized to be superior to another. Non-inferiority trials are used to determine whether a new treatment is no worse than a previous intervention. Equivalence trials are designed to test that two interventions are no better than each other.

A placebo is used to try to avoid a false effect

A well-designed RCT will often use a placebo. The word 'placebo' literally means in Latin 'I will please', and is used so that a participant in a study is unaware whether the intervention is real or not. A placebo may be a pill, cream, injection, acupuncture or any procedure. Often drug intervention RCTs use replica tablets, they don't contain the active ingredient, and these are given out to the participants in the control group.

Box 3.13 describes how a study used sham acupuncture as a placebo. Even the clinician may be seen as a placebo, as positive words of encouragement may be better than no words at all. The acupuncture trial gave for one control group the full experience of sitting with an acupuncturist. The only difference was that the needles were not located in the same places an acupuncturist would use.

A placebo is used to avoid the placebo effect in the study. This effect is where a substance or procedure may have an effect, positive or negative, on the outcome studied, where it should objectively have no such effect. There is disagreement over the roots of the discovery of the placebo effect. One of the most interesting is where a nurse in World War II, on finding that morphine was nearly depleted, prepared a soldier for surgery by injecting him with a water solution. The soldier thought this was a strong analgesic, and went on to have surgery and not fall into shock.

The way in which the placebo effect operates is open to debate, but some scientists have proposed that there is real physiological response, such as reducing the sensation of pain, due to the brain being coerced into believing in an intervention, even when it is inert (Moerman and Jonas, 2002).

The placebo effect may even be used as a treatment in itself. Placebo drugs have been developed and used by physicians, an example being 'Obecalp': the word placebo written backwards. These inert tablets may be used to convince a patient they are being treated with a pharmaceutical. The effect may be enhanced by having grades of Obecalp, so that a large tablet that is difficult to swallow may be perceived as even better than a 'standard' placebo.

In contrast to these there is the 'nocebo', which comes from the Latin 'I will harm'. This is where a person receives harmful, unpleasant or undesirable responses to an inert drug. These responses are not due to any real action, but due to the participant's expectation of a pessimistic or negative outcome.

Blinding is used to avoid bias

A study often uses 'blinding', or 'masking', to improve the design, and this forms best practice in the implementation of drug trials. In a blinded study the nature of the intervention, either as a real or true intervention, or some sort of sham intervention or none at all, is not shared with participants in the study.

Blinding refers to the practice of not informing a person about the allocation of a study participant into the control or intervention arm. A traditional naming of single-, double-, or even triple-blinded has been used. But this may be misleading as it is not clear which person is not receiving the information about the allocation of the intervention. Through common usage, in a single-blinded study the participant will generally be unaware of their allocation. In our example (Box 3.13) the researchers went to great lengths to single-blind their study. One arm was given true acupuncture, whilst a second arm received sham acupuncture where the needles were not inserted where Chinese medicine determined. In most drug trials, it is only necessary to use a placebo drug to implement single blinding.

In a double-blinded trial the treating clinicians also do not know whether the participant is allocated to the treatment or control arm. This means that a clinician or healthcare professional treating a patient should not differ in their approach in any way between control and active treatment groups. Blinding is 'broken' at the end for the analysis, so that the study results can be examined properly. It is not always feasible to either single or double-blind. In the acupuncture trial (Box 3.13), the acupuncturists had to know which group the patient was in, so they could implement the sham acupuncture where necessary.

There is also a growing use of triple-blinded trials, where the person who then measures the response to the intervention, and then does the analysis, is unaware of the true allocation until the analysis is complete. The analysts will, of course, know that there are at least two groups, but will not be aware of whether they are in an active intervention group or control group. A trial may be 'unblinded', or open-label, where no attempt is made to mask the allocation of treatment from all participants, care-givers and those assessing outcomes.

Analysis provides a relative risk

At its simplest, the analysis of an RCT provides a relative risk for developing the outcome comparing the intervention to controls. To begin we calculate the event rates, or rates of the outcome, in the exposed (EER) and unexposed (UER) groups as

$$EER = \frac{e_1}{e_0 + e_1}$$

and

$$UER = \frac{u_1}{u_0 + u_1}$$

where e_1 and e_0 are the number of events and non-events in the intervention group or exposed group, and u_1 and u_0 are the number of events and non-events in the control group respectively. The relative risk (RR) is the ratio of these two event rates:

$$RR = \frac{EER}{UER}$$

Using an example to illustrate this, a group of researchers published an RCT of the use of aspirin and antioxidants to prevent death from coronary heart disease and stroke (Belch *et al.*, 2008). The trial randomized 1276 adults in total aged 40 or over with diabetes and an ankle brachial pressure index of 0.99 or less but with no symptomatic cardiovascular disease. There were four arms, and we report here the number of participants in the intervention arm which received aspirin and the control arm which received no active pharmaceuticals as part of the trial (Table 3.1).

Table 3.1. Results from the aspirin trial (Belch *et al.*, 2008).

| | Number of participants | |
	Intervention group	Control group
Event: death	38	42
Non-event: alive	280	276
Total	318	318

The death rate, which is the event rate in the two groups, exposed to the intervention and unexposed, is

$$EER = \frac{38}{280 + 38} = 0.119$$

and

$$UER = \frac{42}{276 + 42} = 0.132$$

This shows that the death rate, over the course of the trial, in the unexposed or control groups was approximately 13%, and in the intervention group was lower at 12%. The relative risk of death in the intervention group compared to the control group is

$$RR = \frac{0.119}{0.132} = 0.90$$

This suggests that there is a decreased risk of death in the intervention (aspirin) group compared to the group not taking aspirin.

Analysis is best performed as intention to treat

When an RCT is performed, it is very rare for every participant to complete and adhere correctly to their treatment regime. This includes both those in the control and treatment groups. The drop-out may be for a variety of reasons, such as the patients cannot tolerate the drugs, or a therapy is unpleasant or too time-consuming. Participants might perceive their treatment as being ineffective or a waste of their time and choose to take other medication.

This has relevance for the way in which the data is analysed. If you were to restrict the analysis to only those who completed their treatments this will skew the results and will not represent real-life scenarios. To replicate a more realistic situation, the data is analysed using the initial group assignments, regardless of whether the participants continued their treatment or not. Where participants were initially chosen as controls, they are retained as controls and where participants were in the active treatment group the analysis is done that way, regardless of where the participants ended up.

This is known as an intention-to-treat (ITT) analysis and is best practice for the conduct and analysis of RCTs. In a more technical sense, using the treatment that a participant is on at the end of the trial is the same as breaking the randomization.

In the aspirin example (Table 3.1) it is likely that some of those taking aspirin may have stopped due to side-effects of taking the drug. Gastrointestinal symptoms are likely to have been experienced by some in the intervention arm. These people may have stopped taking the tablets, but the analysis was conducted using ITT.

Number needed to treat or harm

A statistic that is often reported is the number of people that are needed to be treated using the active treatment, to prevent a single episode of the outcome we are interested in. This is known as number needed to treat (NNT). When the intervention is harmful leading to some unintended side effect, or when we are interested in removing the risk factor to prevent an outcome, then the number needed to harm (NNH) may be reported. The ideal NNT has a value of one, where all people improve with the intervention and nobody improves in the control group.

The NNT is calculated as the inverse of the absolute risk reduction (ARR; see Section 4.7 for definition and calculation)

$$NNT = \frac{1}{ARR}$$

It is a 'natural number', in that it uses whole integers to express something, rather than fractions which are more difficult and less accessible for clinicians, scientists and the public. Returning to the example of preventing deaths using aspirin in people with diabetes (Table 3.1 and Section 4.7) the number needed to treat is:

$$NNT = \frac{1}{0.013} = 76.9$$

This tells us that we must treat 77 people with aspirin to prevent one death in this group of people. This is an important measure for health economists and politicians as it tells us what level of spending will be needed to achieve health benefits.

Conduct and reporting of RCTs is carefully monitored

The conduct of RCTs is monitored for adherence to clinical and research governance, such as informed consent of the participants. It is usual for a data monitoring committee to check that recruitment is proceeding at a satisfactory pace. Our study example of aspirin and coronary heart disease found that their recruitment was slower than expected. The data monitoring and ethics committee were involved in approving the continuation of the study.

Trials may also employ 'stopping rules' where suspension of a trial may occur when certain conditions are met. These are often associated with either serious side-effects from the intervention, or where there are clear differences between the control arm and intervention arm. It may be deemed unethical to continue in this situation. However, there is controversy in this approach, as the study may not, if completed, show such an effect. It is clear that the stopping of a trial should be done only when there is compelling statistical support for this and there has been a sufficient recruitment of participants. Other stopping rules may be employed when new, external evidence suggests that there is no need to continue the trial, or where the trial participants are showing no significant differences between the control and intervention groups.

In 1996 a statement was published, known as Consolidated Standards of Reporting Trials (CONSORT), which recommends a minimum set of standards when publishing and reporting clinical trials in medicine. CONSORT came out of two groups, working independently, both with the aim to improve the way trials were reported and therefore conducted. Over 600 journals now are signed up to CONSORT, including many of the world's most important such as *The Lancet* and *JAMA*. Since 1996, two further refined and more detailed statements have been made, in 2001 and 2010. CONSORT extensions have been developed to take into account more elaborate and complicated RCT designs.

Drug trials are divided into phases

With respect to trials of drugs, the process for getting full approval for a drug to be used by a health service involves many phases. The phases are not all randomized controlled trials; indeed only one phase (phase 3) is necessarily of this design. Before clinical trials occur, there is a substantial pre-clinical phase involving in-vitro and animal testing. Once the drug is deemed suitable for use in humans the process follows:

Phase 0, referred to as 'first-in-human' trials, where very small doses of the drug of interest are given to a small number of people, commonly 10–15. The doses are calculated to be below any therapeutic effect and participants are monitored to ensure that the drug and the body are behaving how the early pre-clinical testing would predict.
Phase 1, where a small group, typically around 20–100, of healthy volunteers are given the drug. Dose escalation is used to check for levels of safety, and that the drug is working in the way predicted.
Phase 2, where a larger group of volunteers, often again healthy, are tested for the efficacy of the drug that the body responds in a therapeutic way without undesirable toxic effects.
Phase 3, the first time a true RCT is used to test the ability of the drug to treat the disease of interest. After successful completion of phase 3 trials, the drug is usually given a licence and marketed for use.
Phase 4, post-marketing trials to check on continued safety and efficacy.

Strengths and weaknesses of RCT designs

In the range of epidemiological study designs, the RCT provides strong evidence for the role of a potential intervention. This may be for the cause of a disease or an intervention for prevention of a disease. The experimental nature of the design, where the researcher intervenes and assigns people to groups, is a major strength. The randomized nature of the assignment, allowing the researcher no role in the assignment of participants to treatment or control groups, leads to the design being considered free from confounding bias.

The design is not free from selection bias. The epidemiologists must work with whoever agrees to participate; this group may not represent the base population that the scientist intends to investigate. The scientist must examine their group of participants, to see how closely they represent the populations, and interpret their results accordingly. For example, were the study participants who took part a different age profile to the original group selected, then the analyst must make the reader aware of this. This is a problem potentially for external validity. The ITT analysis approach is intended to deal to some extent with the issues of adhering to the intervention.

In 1950, a scientist re-analysed some old experiments from the Hawthorne Works, a Western Electric factory in the United States. Landsberger showed that people may modify or improve their behaviours just by the very fact that they are being studied by science. This is known as the Hawthorne effect, and needs to be borne in mind when designing and analysing a study. This is not exactly the same as the placebo effect.

The RCT is inappropriate for many issues and diseases that need to be studied. This may be due to the high cost of an intervention study, as RCTs can be prohibitively expensive. Or, more likely, this is because the experimental manipulation of the intervention is unethical. This is most common for interventions with putative risk factors for disease. This was illustrated by a sarcastic article in *BMJ* (Smith and Pell, 2003) reporting on a search of the literature for RCTs that examined the effectiveness of the parachute in avoiding death due to 'gravitational challenge'. Many things are beyond the need for science to examine, as the control group in this example would all be given a placebo parachute and would die. This is unethical and would never be conducted.

Summary

The randomized controlled trial, known as the RCT, is as close as you can get to an experimental study design within the constraints of human medical research. For this reason RCTs are considered to be the best approach to testing new interventions. Indeed, all new drugs must usually go through an RCT to show that they are effective. The design examines the efficacy of an intervention, to prevent a disease, or to test a therapeutic for an existing disease.

Participants are randomly assigned to the active treatment group or a control group, and followed up to assess the rate of the outcome in these groups. There are other features of RCTs which improve their implementation. This includes blinding, which is employed to make sure that reporting from the patient and researchers is not biased by the group allocation. Single blinding is where only one group of people are unaware of the allocation. This is usually, in practice, the patient. Double blinding is where both the patient and the treating clinicians or researchers are unaware of the group allocation.

A placebo is an important way to ensure the patients and/or clinicians are unaware of the group allocation. This can take many forms. The most common is to give the participants in the control arm a tablet with no active ingredient, which is identical in look and taste to the real drug. Or, for other interventions, a more elaborate placebo may be employed. For example, sham acupuncture can be used to make the patient believe they are receiving real acupuncture.

An intention-to-treat analysis is used by researchers to ensure that the results are as generalizable as possible. They reflect what may happen in real life when an intervention is used. For example, where a drug treatment has many unwanted side-effects, then this form of analysis will replicate those conditions.

The relative risk, and more usefully the relative risk reduction and numbers needed to treat or harm, are the measures used to define the strength of the intervention on the outcome.

Self-test questions

Q 3.8.1: In an experiment to compare two treatments, subjects are allocated at random so that:
A The experimenter will not know which treatment the subjects receive
B The sample refers to a known population
C The subjects get the treatment best suited to them
D The two groups will be as similar as possible, apart from treatment

Q 3.8.2: For randomized controlled trials which of the following statements is correct?
A In a single-blind trial, patients will not know if they are in the treatment group or the control group
B Patients are always able to give informed consent before recruitment into an RCT
C Patients who do not complete the course must be excluded from the analysis

Q 3.8.3: Randomized controlled trials are better than case series as a means to measure effectiveness because:
A All patients are included in RCTs
B All RCTs are published
C Patients never know whether they have received active treatment or placebo
D RCTs deal with both known and unknown confounding factors

Q 3.8.4: Randomized controlled trials:
A Are not prone to bias from patients dropping out of the treatment or control group
B Are unethical for life-threatening diseases like cancer
C Have been performed for nearly all common medical interventions
D Produce conclusions which are specific only to the study sample

Q 3.8.5: Intention-to-treat analysis is used because:
A Assessment of treatment adherence is not possible
B It most closely reflects what might be observed in actual practice
C Some people withdraw from the study
D This form of analysis is less complicated than any other form

3.9 Qualitative Research

- Pre-requisite sections: 3.1–3.3.
- Learning outcome: By the end of the section you should be able to describe qualitative research and identify the design in any given study as well as its advantages and disadvantages.

Who, what, when, where and how. We have considered all of these questions in previous sections and now we will pause to discuss a research method that focuses on the why. Qualitative research provides a methodology to answer the issue that Einstein raised: 'Not everything that counts can be counted, and not everything that can be counted counts'.

Starting in anthropology, qualitative research is conducted through the analysis of information which is often, although not exclusively, presented in an unstructured format. Qualitative research uses interview transcripts, open-ended items in survey responses, other forms of text such as emails, written notes and responses from feedback forms, in addition to other forms of media such as photos and videos to attempt to shed light on or indeed answer a research question. In mixed methods research both quantitative and qualitative forms of data are used. We will first focus on qualitative methods before moving to their integration into quantitative methods.

Qualitative research is used to gain an understanding or answer the question as to why people engage in certain behaviours, and not in others. There is qualitative data in many forms, which people may not normally realize contain information (Box 3.14). Qualitative research is an attempt to get access to people's ideas, attitudes, behaviours, value systems, concerns, motivations, aspirations, expectations, culture or lifestyles in ways that are difficult using quantitative research methods.

The outcomes of qualitative research can inform business decisions, policy formation and communication strategies and both provide outcomes for research and generate research ideas and novel methodologies themselves. Focus groups, in-depth interviews, ethnography and project evaluation approaches are the main methods used. Collecting and analysing the information produced by these methods can be difficult and time consuming using manual methods. It is generally inductive, which is the process of inferring a generalized conclusion from particular instances. It is these instances which are the data.

Qualitative research methods can be useful when there is little known on a topic. This can generally arise when particular populations are not given a voice or systematically excluded from research. This can be the case when dealing with sensitive topics such as the attitude of sex workers, or difficult-to-access groups and

---

Box 3.14. Social networking research

There can be many health conditions that affect members of a community, and patients may have specific needs as a direct result of their illness. Some of these will be known about by health authorities, and some less so: the people worst affected by a health condition may not be able to leave their homes to see a doctor, meaning their needs are under-represented in the community or not represented at all. Concerned patients or members of their families may use online social networking to share their stories, detail their experiences and contact others who share their situation. In doing so, they are not only providing discussion and support but also creating records that can be collated to form data. A scientist could do a qualitative analysis of the content of emails, for example, to identify the relative importance of community services such as personal care, paramedical, respite and transport. This in turn could be used to approach the health authority to fund some research into the needs of patients with that condition.

---

subcultures such as the homeless or itinerant populations. Culturally defined experiences are also areas where qualitative research can be useful.

What is the data?

Box 3.15 shows the types of data that are used in qualitative research. We measure these data by assigning codes to what is present in each of these data forms and also what is missing. We are sifting the data, and coding is this process of sifting, identifying and measuring themes, ideas and categories. Once we have established a code we then mark similar passages of text with the same code. This can help us easily retrieve codes, so we can count them, for example, and their attached text so we can assess what they mean. By coding data it is now easier to search, compare and identify patterns.

The codes can be based on themes, topics, ideas, concepts, terms, phrases and keywords. Electronically coding is quite simple as most word processing software has search tools. It can get a little more difficult with sections of an audio or video recording or parts of images; however it is still possible with the right software.

Reliability and validity is an issue with all research methods. In qualitative research internally valid data is known as credible data. This involves the data being seen as credible or believable from the participants' perspective. Remember we are looking to get rich data from the perspective of the participant so these criteria need to seem reasonable. Now we have an opportunity to test how well one coder assigns a code compared to how another coder assigns that same code on that same piece of text.

External validity or generalizability can be considered in terms of how transferable our results are and how representative of other contexts or settings are our findings. Whereas participants are responsible for credibility, researchers are responsible for how transferable the results are. Researchers do this by describing a research context clearly and documenting all assumptions they made in developing these criteria.

Given things in this world change, dependability of our results is important. This relates to the quantitative concept of reliability and the researcher again is responsible

---

Box 3.15. Types of qualitative data

In-depth/unstructured/semi-structured interviews
Structured interview questionnaires containing sections for open comments
Focus groups
Unstructured/structured diaries
Observation field notes
Diagrams/other anthropological material (data relating to the origin, behaviour, and physical, social and cultural development of people)
Case study notes
Meeting minutes
Personal documents (e.g. letters, correspondence)
Press clippings
Photographs or any other type of visual material

---

for describing any changes that occur in a setting and how these changes affected the variables, theme, codes and ultimately the theories and hypothesis under study.

Objectivity is a hallmark of the scientific process. In qualitative research, confirmability refers to the degree to which the results could be confirmed or corroborated by other participants. We could do this by checking and rechecking data throughout the study, comparing codes between researchers. Also the researcher can search for negative instances that contradict prior observations to see if they still hold up.

Codes are labelled in order to provide the coder with an indication of the idea or concept that underpins the theme or category. Any parts of the data that relate to that code are coded with that label. If some text is identified from the data that is important to the research question but does not fit the codes already existing, then a new code is created. As the researcher reads through the data, the number of codes they have will change as more topics or themes become apparent and some become subsumed under broader and more encompassing codes.

Where to begin?

A researcher usually starts coding with themes identified from *a priori* ideas such as theories. A coding framework can be useful here as a way to organize the data as it presents itself within the analysis. Coding frameworks can develop from previous research or theory, the specific research questions you are answering, the questions from the interview schedule, or a hypothesis you may have developed.

Alternatively when new codes emerge from your data set you are using a technique which is a basis for grounded theory. Grounded codes develop from the data when you disregard previous knowledge of the subject and focus on finding new themes and ideas from your data.

Grounded theory

Grounded theory (GT) seems to be anathema to the scientific method. By beginning the research process with data collection, we are not sure what exactly we are testing. However from the data collected, important data are marked with codes, with the codes then grouped into similar concepts and from these concepts, categories are formed. From here we can create a theory which stems directly from the data, not the other way around.

Grounded theory begins within the context we are interested in studying, and the researcher is trying to understand what is happening in this context and how the participants develop and manage their roles. A constant comparison process as defined below is important in GT as the researcher compares data to other initial data collected. This allows a theory to emerge.

Researchers however usually have some codes already in mind and are looking to gain greater insights or investigate new areas which may arise out of the data. Some useful questions to think about when coding data include: What is going on? What are people doing? What is the person saying? What do these actions and statements take for granted? How do structure and context serve to support, maintain, impede or change these actions and statements?

Constant comparison

Constant comparison is a GT approach whereby you code some text and you then compare it with all those passages of text you have already coded. This allows the newly coded text to be coded in a consistent manner with previous text and also ensures that you are double-checking previously coded text. During this process you can also see how the code differs from other codes. These similarities and differences might shed important light on your research question.

The repetition of words might also be useful, and listing the most commonly used words is another data analysis technique. Looking around a specific word for its context can also be a useful technique. Noting the words that are not used also sheds light on issues that may be culturally sensitive or not relevant for a particular population. Similes, metaphors and analogies are often used in everyday language to convey meaning. Searching for examples of these can provide rich insights. Connections between terms such as the causal ('since', 'because', 'as' etc.) or logical ('implies', 'means', 'is one of' etc.) terms can be useful as can assessing any unmarked text to examine themes that may have been missed.

Are we there yet?

In collecting and interpreting data about a particular code, researchers start to see the same pattern repeated over and over again. When the interviews cease adding to what you already know about a category, you cease coding for that category.

Problems and limitations are similar to those for quantitative methods. When there are inadequate amounts of evidence the conclusions of the research do not stand up. Similarly when the variety of evidence is limited you may have a data set that is not generalizable to other contexts. Paying attention to data that is the exception to the category the researcher is investigating is just as important as the mountain of evidence which supports a code or category. These discrepancies help suggest alternative hypotheses that might need examination in and of themselves.

For the researcher, data overload is an oft-quoted problem when using qualitative data analysis. A journal can be helpful for the researcher to place their first impressions in their appropriate context. This, coupled with comparison with other coders, helps increase the likelihood that a conclusion is valid. Missing information can be important and should be reported as such. This is an answer for another piece of research to find. Association does not equal causation and co-occurrences and correlations within qualitative research are a problem and should be kept in mind when it comes to interpreting the data.

Mixed methods

Mixed methods research is defined as any research where both qualitative and quantitative approaches to research are employed in either data collection or data analysis and interpretation phases within a single study, or both. Mixed methods are seen as distinct from the positivist philosophy of quantitative research and the constructivist perspective of qualitative research. Positivism is a theory of knowledge which argues for the use of the research methods. For example in social science and the study of social phenomena it defines social phenomena as having an objective reality and therefore able to be counted. Questions can then be asked as to what is knowledge? How is this knowledge acquired? How do we know what we know?

The constructivist philosophy of qualitative research is different again. Constructivism is a theory where a premise is that social phenomena and the associated meanings are constructed by the people involved in using them or observing them, rather than as objects we can count and that exist independently of the people involved.

Mixed methods are useful for purposes of corroboration (do the results of different methods support each other?), expansion (use of a different method to add to an understanding) or initiation (contrasting methods to develop new ideas and understandings) (Rossman and Wilson, 1985, 1994). We can do these separately, in sequence or in parallel and with one method more dominant than the other, or we can combine them. Caracelli and Greene describe this integration below (Caracelli and Greene, 1997). For example, you might conduct a qualitative study in which you observe the behaviours you are interested in as a participant and also interview people about their attitudes towards this behaviour. Another example is in a quantitative study where you administer an attitude survey to students and also collect information from computer records about the frequency of use of web-based course materials. In other words, you make use of methods that are broadly compatible within a paradigm or a set of beliefs and values.

Summary

There are similarities and differences between qualitative and quantitative methods. As with both methods, qualitative methods should be applied after a careful consideration of 'purpose' and reason for completing a research activity and what is the 'question' you are attempting to answer and providing time for reflection of 'theoretical assumptions'. Qualitative methods need to be systematic, rigorous and planned while maintaining a balance between being strategically conducted, yet flexible and taking into account the contextual issues. Qualitative methods need to involve the type of critical self-scrutiny that is common to the scientific method and able to produce social explanations which are generalizable.

Self-test questions

Q 3.9.1: Which of the following best describes qualitative research?
A Involves statistical analysis
B No preconceived assumptions/hypothesis
C Research question/hypothesis comes first
D The findings are generalizable

Q 3.9.2: Subjectivity is defined as which of the following?
A The strength of quantitative research
B The art of choosing university topics

C The opposite of objectivity

D An inherent flaw of qualitative research

Q 3.9.3: True or false? Quantitative methods:

A Are more rigorous than qualitative

B Are the best method to use when exploring meaning and why questions

C Are the most appropriate method for the new, relatively unskilled researcher

D Are far inferior to qualitative approaches

E Don't need to be underpinned by theory

Q 3.9.4: True or False? Successful interviewing:

A Is about correcting your interviewee

B Asks lots of knowledge questions

C Is where the interviewer talks more than the interviewee

D Is open to the unexpected

E Is where the interviewer is non-judgemental

3.10   A Hierarchy of Evidence

- Pre-requisite sections: 3.2–3.8.
- Learning outcome: By the end of the section you should be able to describe the relative merits of different epidemiological study designs.

The world of medical science, epidemiology and clinical research is expanding at ever-increasing rates, meaning for any clinician or scientist it is difficult to assess the whole portfolio of evidence. For example PubMed, a free online database provided by United States National Library of Medicine at the National Institutes of Health, comprises more than 20,000,000 citations for biomedical literature from Medline, life science journals and online books and points of entry (for example, Google Scholar), leaving any researcher easily overwhelmed.

Evidence-based medicine is 'the conscientious, explicit, and judicious use of current best evidence in making decisions about the care of individual patients. The practice of evidence-based medicine … means integrating individual clinical expertise with the best available external clinical evidence from systematic research.' (Sackett *et al.*, 1996). From this it is clear that an evidence-based practitioner must be able to decide which, of the colossal amount of published research, is the best evidence. This approach must also be expanded to evidence-based practice for care of populations, using public health to protect the health of groups of people.

A practitioner's approach may be informal and subjective

A single healthcare practitioner, when faced with a clinical or public health problem, may:

- Search for guidelines, such as those provided by UK National Institute for Health and Clinical Evidence (NICE), or other more specialized organizations such as the British Hypertension Society.
- If no guidelines are available or suitable, do a quick search on Medline, GP

Notebook, Patient UK or Medscape. A systematic review may be available, such as those provided by Cochrane.

● Based on the abstracts and articles, identify rapidly the most relevant and strongest studies.
● Synthesize their findings and recommendations.
● Integrate it with clinical expertise and the patients' circumstances, values and preferences.

The process is quick, very informal and usually far from systematic. Most practitioners might take a short-cut to the end result by first talking with a colleague, who may or may not have broad experience or have recently done a similar trawl of the literature. When groups of clinicians work together they often develop materials that are of benefit to those who lack the time to complete the above. Interestingly this is the basis for some English law on medical negligence cases. The Bolam test states that using expert opinion is important for determining the appropriateness of clinical decisions.

Healthcare is not universally evidence-based

The randomized controlled trial, abbreviated to RCT, is a cornerstone of evidence-based medicine; however, it is not universally applied to interventions. Only 40% of surgical issues may be addressed by RCTs (Solomon and McLeod, 1995) with only about 5–10% of surgical scientific literature reporting RCTs (Slim, 2005). The RCT is even less suited to providing evidence for other interests, such as preventive measures.

Transferring scientific evidence into clinical practice is difficult, as clinicians are reluctant; guidelines, although having a long history and regularly updated, are implemented in an *ad-hoc* manner (for example in colorectal cancer (Bampton *et al.*, 2007)). Implementation of guidelines is a difficult process taking time (Grol, 2001; Antes *et al.*, 2006; Forbes *et al.*, 2008; Hardman and Carlson, 2008) and there is variation between countries (Lassen *et al.*, 2005).

It has been claimed only 10–20% of medical decisions are based on scientific evidence (Slim *et al.*, 2004) although this is disputed (Howes *et al.*, 1997). To illustrate this: cancer is a leading cause of premature death. Medical knowledge is thought to be sufficient that one third of cancers could be prevented, one third cured given early diagnosis, and the remainder treated (WHO, 2006).

Continuing medical education is still delivered in traditional and generally passive formats with variable effect on practice (Young *et al.*, 2006). Clinicians are not good at evaluating their own knowledge or clinical skill (Davis *et al.*, 2006). For example evaluation of performance on 439 quality indicators for 30 conditions found 55% of patients in the US received recommended care, with no difference across preventive, acute or chronic care (McGlynn *et al.*, 2003).

A systematic approach is needed

To overcome a lack of a systematic approach the practitioner may use explicit, transparent methods to assess the results in published research, applying rules of evidence to establish internal validity, how much a piece of research adheres to reporting standards and how generalizable the results are. From this we find some pieces of evidence more robust than others and we can develop a hierarchy which is an arrangement of items whose research methods are represented as 'above', 'below' or 'at the same level as' one another. The quality of research is partly due to the design of the study and through repeated analyses of study design we know that some designs are more useful than others. From this a hierarchy has been developed.

Many different authors have produced different versions of a 'hierarchy of evidence' with respect to study design. Study designs can be categorized in a number of ways, one way is to look at what the study can provide. A descriptive analysis will describe the number of cases in a population. It might also be able to look at the time, place and person of cases. Most other designs allow analytical epidemiology to be conducted, where a risk factor can be examined in relation to the incidence of a disease. This will hopefully give a clearer clue as to the relationship that factor has with the disease. Analytical study designs are placed higher on the hierarchy than those that are merely descriptive.

Another way to examine the study designs is to classify as either observational, where the researcher is entirely passive in the disease process, or experimental, such as the RCT design. In this, the researcher actively intervenes to modify the conditions that participants experience. Again, the experimental study designs are at the top of the hierarchy. Observational designs are lower on the hierarchy.

One hierarchy of evidence

We will be taking a look at one version of the hierarchy of evidence, of which there are many different versions. Of course, this does not mean that we can avoid all of the other issues surrounding the way a study is conducted. A poorly conducted study will give poor results, regardless of its place on the hierarchy.

Taking a look at the hierarchy (Fig. 3.4), at the bottom of the figure is the anecdote. This is the least good form of epidemiological evidence, prone to the vagaries of subjective opinion and hidden agendas. Next, the case report, which is a report of a particularly interesting case published in the literature. A case series is a collection of such case reports on a specific subject. For example, a case series of Kaposi's sarcoma was reported amongst young gay men in New York in the early 1980s. This is of interest since Kaposi's sarcoma was rare and only occurred in older people, and became, with hindsight, one of the first indications of the existence of AIDS.

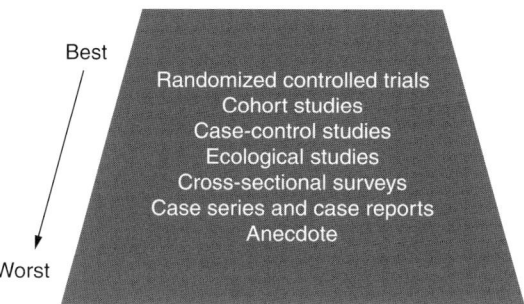

Fig. 3.4. Hierarchy of evidence.

Next up is the cross-sectional survey that measures the current health status of a population. The prevalence measured within the survey can then be used to infer prevalence in the population. It is not very useful for looking at associations between risk factors and outcomes, and for this reason lies near to the bottom of the hierarchy. An ecological study uses measurements taken at the population level in order to assess the influence of a risk factor. This is still near the bottom because of the possibility of bias due to the ecological fallacy.

We now move to studies that measure and examine individuals. In a case-control study people are selected on the basis of whether they do or do not have a particular disease under study, making these studies retrospective. The groups are compared with respect to the proportion having a history of an exposure or characteristic of interest. A cohort is a group of people sharing a characteristic. For example, all people born in 1945, which is known as a birth cohort, or pregnant women who had an abdominal X-ray during their first trimester. Cohort studies are usually prospective, which is before the disease develops, but they can be undertaken retrospectively. The researcher 'follows' groups with different exposures to a risk factor, to record the incidence of disease in each group.

A randomized controlled trial is a planned experiment involving patients and designed to discover the most appropriate intervention for future patients with a given medical condition, or to prevent a given disease. This experimental design is considered as one of the strongest forms of evidence for epidemiology.

Meta-analysis is a method to combine the results of several studies. We have not placed this study on the hierarchy; this is because the meta-analysis is only as good as the studies that it combines. So, a meta-analysis of ecological studies may not provide as good evidence as a single RCT.

Hierarchies are limited by what they assess

A limitation of hierarchies is that many focus mainly on effectiveness. Effectiveness is whether an intervention works as intended. However, one can also focus on appropriateness, which relates to psychosocial aspects of the intervention and assesses impact on a person, whether this is tolerated by the person and in many cases whether a person would use an intervention. Feasibility is also important as the impact of an intervention on an organization or provider, the resources required to make it happen, may determine whether an intervention is able to be used or implemented at all.

Economists, for example, might be more concerned with spillover and scale effects when moving from a small piece of research to a larger scale study. It might be better to be able to supplement evidence from both a randomized trial and a natural experiment. More recent and those pieces of research published in more high-ranking journals may also be considered to have greater weight and importance.

Official agencies have designed hierarchies

Different countries use different hierarchies. The government of the United States of America has designed a hierarchy of evidence from medical research. The best form of evidence is at the top of the hierarchy:

I: Properly powered and conducted randomized controlled trial (RCT); well conducted systematic review or meta-analysis of homogeneous RCTs

II-1: Well-designed controlled trial without randomization

II-2: Well-designed cohort or case-control analytic study

II-3: Multiple time series with or without the intervention; dramatic results from uncontrolled experiments

III: Opinions of respected authorities, based on clinical experience; descriptive studies or case reports; reports of expert committees

The government of the United Kingdom has developed an evidence hierarchy for those making policy (Social Exclusion Task Force, 2008):

1. Systematic review – Synthesis of results from several studies
2. Randomized controlled trial – Population allocated randomly to groups
3. Quasi-experimental study – Similar populations compared
4. Pre-post study – Results compared before and after intervention.

Summary

A clinician or public health practitioner must use the best evidence that is available to them. There are many thousands of articles published each year and it is exceptionally difficult for any one person to quickly synthesize the evidence. But this is a necessary step in evidence-based practice.

One way to rapidly determine the most appropriate studies that should be integrated into practice is to use a hierarchy of evidence. Any one hierarchy may be based on different strengths that a study design brings to the research question. We have presented one hierarchy that places the lowest form of quality of evidence as the anecdote, moving through the different study designs on to the RCT, which is considered as the strongest form of evidence. This is because the experimental design of the RCT is more powerful than the observational study designs lower down on the hierarchy.

Finally the practitioner must not ignore other assessments of any one study design, such as the size of the participant group, or the bias and error associated with different study designs.

Self-test questions

Q 3.10.1: True or false? Observational studies are superior to experimental studies.

Q 3.10.2: In considering the 'hierarchy' of study design which of the following is true?
A Cohort studies are superior to case-control studies
B Ecological studies are superior to RCTs
C Cross-sectional surveys are superior to cohort studies
D Case-control studies are superior to RCTs

Q 3.10.3: Which of the following study designs are NOT normally retrospective?
A Case-control

B Cohort

C Ecological

Q 3.10.4: In order to assess how strongly an exposure is associated with a disease, which would be the most relevant health statistic?

A Incidence of the disease among the exposed

B Prevalence of the disease among the exposed

C Prevalence of the exposure

D Relative risk

Q 3.10.5: Which of the following statements about randomized control trials and cohort studies are correct?

A RCTs are more likely to be susceptible to bias

B Only cohort studies permit direct determination of incidence rates

C RCTs have the advantage that the data is readily at hand

D Cohort studies are often used to elucidate factors related to rare diseases

3.11 Systematic Review and Meta-Analysis

- Pre-requisite sections: 3.2–3.9.
- Learning outcome: By the end of the section you should be able to describe systematic reviews, meta-analysis and the relative merits of each.

There are significant areas of knowledge and practice that exist outside the evidence base. Firstly, there may be no evidence, or insufficient evidence, to support clinical decisions in a particular area. For example, we do not know the long-term effects of a newly developed drug when taken for a number of years. Secondly, the evidence base may exist, but we have not put it into practice. This was elegantly summarized by Archie Cochrane in 1971: 'It is surely a great criticism of our profession that we have not organised a critical summary, by speciality or subspecialty, adapted periodically, of all relevant randomised controlled trials.' In this section we will assume the second is true and the evidence exists. We will describe ways in which researchers have attempted to sort the 'wheat from the chaff' and identify what is the best way of delivering evidence-based practice.

Systematic reviews are different to meta-analyses

Decisions about treatment choices should be based on reliable information. But most clinicians are confronted with too much information, in too little time to digest and integrate into their practice. Clinicians are often overwhelmed by the amount of new information and although reviews can efficiently bring clinicians up to date, there are limitations.

We have discussed how research is susceptible to bias and error, even when done by experts. We are trying to avoid the results of a study systematically deviating from the truth, which can appear in the data collection, appraisal and summarizing stage of a review.

A systematic review is done by a panel of experts to survey the state of knowledge at that point in time. Box 3.16 gives some of the stages in conducting a systematic review. Systematic reviews aim to minimize bias and error in a number of ways. Firstly, by having at least two reviewers you are able to measure the level of agreement both between the reviewers and over time for individual reviewers. Secondly, as with the scientific method, you look to inform others as to what you are going to do, before you do it. By publishing a protocol for the systematic review method you are able to allow others to reproduce your work and also allow others to critique the processes you used. These transparent methods are the basis of good science.

A meta-analysis is a process by which results are extracted from individual studies and combined to calculate an overall estimate. This involves carefully determining whether it is appropriate for a series of studies to be combined and whether the result is reliable.

A systematic review does not have to contain a meta-analysis, and similarly a meta-analysis does not have to be based on a systematic review. However, it is common for both to be done simultaneously.

Systematic reviews begin by defining the question

Before embarking on the pile of journal articles, a systematic review needs to define the question under study. What specific intervention are you interested in? In healthcare, we are looking to provide a treatment to improve health which can include medical procedures, applications or services used to try and improve health. We must first define all aspects of treatment and the context in which it occurs.

At first we must locate all the studies that address the question we are interested in. This includes online services like PubMed which comprises over 20,000,000 citations for biomedical literature. Given that these citations and abstracts can include medicine, nursing, dentistry, veterinary medicine, the healthcare system and preclinical sciences, it is essential that we be as specific as possible when using the search parameters.

Box 3.16. A systematic review collates the evidence (http://www.cochrane-handbook.org)

A systematic review attempts to collate all empirical evidence that fits pre-specified eligibility criteria (Antman *et al.*, 1992). The key characteristics of a systematic review are:

- a clearly stated set of objectives with pre-defined eligibility criteria for studies;
- an explicit, reproducible methodology;
- a systematic search that attempts to identify all studies that would meet the eligibility criteria;
- an assessment of the validity of the findings of the included studies, for example through the assessment of risk of bias; and
- a systematic presentation, and synthesis, of the characteristics and findings of the included studies.

The review assesses the quality of the studies

We must define the study subjects, and whether they differ in terms of gender, age and other demographic characteristics. What are the outcomes measured and how are they measured? It is important to determine whether they are a direct measure, self-reported measure or observer-identified measure.

The next stage is to assess whether the studies meet set criteria that may also include other reports, grey literature and unpublished results, usually obtained by direct correspondence with the authors conducting the research. Grey literature is a term used by many librarians and research professionals to mean a body of materials that cannot be found easily through conventional channels such as online databases such as PubMed. The next stages include calculating the results of each study if this has not been completed already by the authors and combining these between studies if appropriate.

The Cochrane Collaboration organizes systematic reviews

It is a huge endeavour to produce systematic reviews and one organization has made it their goal to complete this task. The Cochrane Collaboration is an international network of individuals who voluntarily 'prepare, maintain and promote the accessibility of systematic reviews of the effects of health care interventions'. It is organized around 12 Cochrane Centres and by speciality with over 50 review groups. Their output is considerable; the collaboration produces 300 new reviews per year and updates reviews on a 2–3 year cycle.

The Cochrane Library is a collection of six databases that contain types of evidence with the aim to inform healthcare decision making. These include: Cochrane Database of Systematic Reviews; Cochrane Central Register of Controlled Trials; Cochrane Methodology Register; Database of Abstracts of Reviews of Effects; Health Technology Assessment Database; NHS Economic Evaluation Database.

Meta-analysis summarizes results together

Meta-analysis is the use of statistical methods to summarize the results of independent studies and is achieved by combining information from all studies on a given topic. A meta-analysis can provide a more precise estimate of the effects of a healthcare intervention than those derived from the individual studies included within a review. This is a way to calculate an average estimate providing an 'average' or 'common' effect and statistically combines results from two or more separate studies.

A meta-analysis can allow an investigation of the consistency of evidence across studies, and the exploration of differences between studies. Given that many individual studies are too small to detect important effects, we may combine several studies thereby increasing our chance of detecting an effect. The meta-analysis also allows us to improve the precision of the outcome.

Meta-analyses allow us to settle many controversies arising from conflicting studies or provide a process to generate new hypotheses. The amount of disagreement can be assessed, and the reasons for different results can be explored and in many cases quantified. By improving our precision of the estimate we can also quantify the effect sizes across the studies and also their uncertainty. Investigating consistency of results across variables such as year the study was conducted can also be illuminating. Older studies may have shown a greater effect when compared to more recent studies posing the additional question as to whether the rigour of the studies has improved over time.

Meta-analysis must ensure that studies are not too different

We need to ensure there are no major differences in the study characteristics in such variables as the participants under study, the type of interventions being investigated or the outcomes of each piece of research. When the outcome and treatment effect have been measured in a similar way, it is possible then to compare studies.

The steps involved in doing a meta-analysis require the researchers to define the comparisons for review, decide on the appropriate study results and outcomes for each comparison and select an appropriate summary statistic for each comparison. This last point depends on the type of data you collect. To calculate a single summary statistic to represent the effect found in each study for binary data we need to have the ratio of risks (relative risk), difference in risks (risk difference) or ratio of odds (odds ratio). With continuous data we are interested in the difference between means.

When calculating the difference we are averaging studies and a simple average gives each study an equal weight. This is problematic as some studies are more likely to give an answer closer to the 'true' effect than others given the rigour of their differing methodologies. When we want to weight studies our guiding principle is to give more weight to the studies which give us more information, those that have more participants, more outcomes or events of interest, and lower variance. Weight is proportional to the inverse of the variance as we are more certain of the estimate provided with lower variances.

The results can be assessed through an informal inspection or a formal test. Further, we are able to conduct subgroup analyses when we suspect *a priori* that certain features may influence the effect of an intervention. Sensitivity analysis allows us to question whether the result changes according to small variations in the data and methods used. The choice of treatment effects or method for pooling is also important as are the inclusion and exclusion criteria used to deal with dubious or other data not deemed relevant by the original researchers.

An important bias in the interpretation of meta-analytic data is publication bias. Publication bias is where factors such as whether the article was written in English or reported positive results significantly influence whether the research makes it into the public domain or not.

Summary

The Cochrane Collaboration is one of the best known and respected examples of systematic reviews. Like other collections of systematic reviews, it requires authors to provide a detailed and repeatable plan of their literature search and evaluations of the evidence. Once all the best evidence is assessed, treatment is categorized as 'likely to be beneficial', 'likely to be harmful', or 'evidence did not support either benefit or harm'. A 2007 analysis of 1016 systematic reviews from all 50 Cochrane Collaboration Review Groups found that 44% of the reviews concluded that the intervention was 'likely to be beneficial', 7% concluded that the intervention was 'likely to be harmful', and 49% concluded that evidence 'did not support either benefit or harm'. Ninety-six percent recommended further research.

Both systematic reviews and meta-analyses provide an important method for both identifying unanswered questions and providing the most powerful answer to questions which have troubled clinicians for many years. It must be remembered that any review or meta-analysis is only as good as the included studies: garbage in, garbage out.

Self-test questions

Q 3.11.1: What is a meta-analysis?
A A collection of all studies on a subject
B A combined analysis of all studies on a subject
C A combined analysis of all studies that can be put together on a subject

Q 3.11.2: True or false? A systematic review must contain a meta-analysis.

Q 3.11.3: Which of the following statements is correct in the assessment of published evidence on clinical effectiveness?
A Meta-analysis is sometimes used to combine results of a number of studies
B Only meta-analysis is used for assessing clinical evidence
C Publication bias is not a problem
D Systematic review only uses data from randomized controlled trials

3.12   An Answer From Epidemiology

- Pre-requisite sections: 3.1–3.11.
- Learning outcome: By the end of the section you should be able to describe an example of a disease that can now be prevented.

In Section 3.1 we described cervical cancer, highlighting its role in the deaths of many hundreds of thousands of women globally. There had been major advances in treatment, and in detecting early signs of the disease. However, until the late 1990s, there was no way to prevent the disease.

This is not a 'straw man': with hindsight the solution to the causes of cervical cancer may seem obvious, but they were not. There was a series of confusing and sometimes contradictory pieces of evidence. Its history highlights many important aspects of the ability of epidemiology to prevent disease and death (see Box 3.17.)

Box 3.17. Breakthroughs and straw men

The discovery that cervical cancer can be prevented by a vaccine was a major break-through. Another major success of epidemiology is the smoking ban. Looking back from our vantage point in the present, it can seem hard to believe that everyone didn't always know that smoking was bad for you – how could anyone think that inhaling smoke was not going to damage your health? It can have the appearance of being a 'straw man': an American term to describe a situation that is easy to destroy or contra-dict, like how something made of straw is simple to knock over. Studies into smoking-related disease were not a straw man, however. Looking back to the early part of the twentieth century, smoking was thought to be harmless. Society forgets these things quickly. Although creating a straw man is not technically a violation of the scientific method, it can bring science into disrepute because people see questions that have 'obvious' answers.

An early anecdote pointed the way

It is interesting to note that an early investigation into the possible causes of cervical cancer has become an anecdote. Epidemiology considers this to be one of the least rigorous forms of evidence. But an Italian physician is reported as saying that cervical cancer was far less prevalent in nuns than other women. And his work has been quoted in many dozens of research papers since its publication. This may point to a number of possible risk factors, but sexual activity is now known to be the correct one. Comparing nuns with prostitutes was on the right track – but some interpreted these findings to do with the wearing of corsets.

Epidemiologists got closer to identifying a cause in the mid-20th century

During the 1950s the prevailing thinking was that the cancer was caused by some-thing to do with sexual intercourse, and the herpes virus was implicated. During the 1960s further ecological studies suggested that nuns were indeed at a lower risk of death from cancer of the cervix than other women (Fraumeni *et al.*, 1969). This seemed to tally with the earlier anecdote-driven research findings. However, a puta-tive factor was not identified.

During the 1980s, a case-control study continued to suggest that sexual inter-course was associated with cervical cancer. These studies were able to examine more closely potential risk factors, such as the number of sexual partners and condom use. The researchers discovered that the greater the number of sexual partners, the greater the risk for cervical cancer.

Human papillomavirus was discovered in 1956

Meanwhile, in laboratories, the human papillomavirus, abbreviated to HPV, was discovered in 1956. It was linked to cancer of the skin, and produces warts on the skin. As early as 1976, Harald zur Hausen hypothesized in the scientific literature that HPV plays a role in the aetiology of cervical cancer. In 1983 and 1984, zur Hausen and his collaborators identified HPV16 and HPV18 in precursor lesions for genital cancer and cervical cancer.

Nearly all tissue samples from cervical cancers contain HPV DNA. However, at this point, it was unclear whether this was due to 'reverse causality'. This would be where the cancer leads to increased risk of HPV invasion.

Preventative vaccines were developed against HPV

Vaccines have been developed to prevent HPV. These are effective in protecting against cervical lesions due to HPV16 and 18, and Gardasil® also protects against HPV6 and 11, which are responsible for 90% of genital warts. HPV16 and 18 are responsible for 70% of cervical cancer worldwide. Clinical trials have shown that vaccination reduced the number of people with lesions by 18%. Following these successes many countries are introducing vaccination campaigns against HPV. Some important questions remain, such as how long the protection may be for and vaccination policies, for example whether to vaccinate males also.

The vaccines prevent nearly 100% of the precancerous cervical cell changes caused by HPV for up to 4 years after vaccination among women who were not infected at the time of vaccination. The length of immunity is usually not known when a vaccine is first introduced. Studies have shown people are still protected after five years. More research is required on how long protection will last, and if a booster dose is useful.

Up to half of men in the population may be infected with HPV and the case for vaccinating boys against HPV can be made. Economic considerations are important here as the various strains of HPV also cause anal, penile, head and neck cancers and vaccinating boys could prevent some of these cancers.

These discoveries led to a Nobel Prize

The Nobel Prize in Physiology of Medicine was given to the German scientist: 'Dr. zur Hausen went against current dogma by postulating that the virus caused cervical cancer,' said the Karolinska Institute in Stockholm, in the statement explaining the reasons for the assignment of the prize. Despite the presentation of the Nobel Prize, which was well deserved, it is obvious that Dr zur Hausen was 'standing on the shoulders of giants'. His work and hypothesizing was critical, but many other researchers contributed to the efforts that allowed these breakthroughs to be made.

Summary

This story demonstrates the importance of epidemiology. We now have the capability to prevent a cancer that still kills many thousands of women globally each year. The introduction of a preventative strategy, first identified through careful epidemiological analyses, has given us the hope to reduce, or even eradicate this form of cancer for women in the future.

Self-test question

Q 3.12.1: Can you think of any other diseases which can be prevented through the work of epidemiology?

Q 3.12.2: A study collects the number of cases per 1000 population of cervical cancer for countries around the world. This is compared with per capita fat consumption, to examine whether fat consumption may cause this cancer. What is the name of this type of study design?
A Ecological study
B Cohort study
C Case-control study
D Case series

Further Reading

Recreational Water Illness Outbreak Response Toolkit. Available at http://www.cdc.gov/healthywater/emergency/toolkit/rwi-outbreak-toolkit.html (accessed 30 September 2012)

4 Dealing With the Numbers

The practice of statistical epidemiology involves collecting information. Much of this is in the form of numbers, quantities that are measured and counted. It is essential that the scientist knows how to deal with the data appropriately. This chapter focuses on the presentation of data that you collect and the way these quantities are analysed.

4.1 Types of Data

- Pre-requisite sections: 1.2.
- Learning outcome: By the end of the section you should be able to identify the type of data that constitutes a variable.

All forms of science, including medical research, generate and rely on data. Data includes observations on something that varies from patient to patient, and when these data are stored and collected into a group this is known as a 'variable'. As an example, the age of patients with a certain disease may be collected and recorded: this forms a variable, it varies between patients. Each person in this study would be an 'observation', or in database parlance a 'record'. It is common to think about the data in a grid, with the rows forming the observations, in this case the patients, and the columns the data fields or variables.

Variables are either dependent or independent, which relates to the process by which the quantities are generated. A dependent variable is caused by some other variable or variables. The variable that causes the dependent variable is the independent variable. In epidemiology, the outcome is often referred to as the dependent variable as it is caused by other quantities. Risk factors, exposures or treatments are often, for this reason, known as the independent variable as they are considered to cause the outcome.

Variables may be qualitative or quantitative

The data that form variables have different characteristics, which we may classify into two main groups. Data that is measured, that creates a number, is quantitative. For example, a measurement of weight is quantitative as it produces a numerical value. In addition, the value will usually have a scale, such as a length in metres, or a weight in kilograms.

Qualitative data, often seen as the opposite of quantitative, is data that is not measured and not usually reported on a scale. For example there have been many studies of eye colour, as it an indicator of a person's susceptibility to ultraviolet radiation in sunlight. The colour of a person's eyes may be measured using techniques

---

developed by colorimetry: the quantification of human colour perception. Anyone who has changed colours of text in word processing software on a computer will be aware of the 'RGB' colour model, where red, green and blue lights combine to create a range of different colours. These may be expressed quantitatively, and the colour of a person's eye may be measured in the same way.

Alternatively, a human observer may classify the colour of the eye, by placing the findings into categories. The findings are based on the subjective opinions of the researcher defining the categories. Eye colour may be classified using standard language, such as 'blue' or 'brown', or with reference to a series of colours on card. Either way, the method relies on a subjective assessment of the colour, which will open the recording of accurate data to many external influences. Influences include the observer's own colour perception, or their unconscious expectations of the eye colour for the ethnic group of the person observed.

Qualitative data may be converted into quantitative data. For example, a record of a conversation is a qualitative piece of information. A researcher may use language analysis to examine the speech patterns. These data may then be converted into quantitative data through counting aspects of the conversation. For example, in a recorded conversation, the researcher could add up the number of times the speaker used the word 'I'. These data would then be a quantitative record of qualitative data.

Qualitative data may be nominal or ordinal

What types of results are anticipated from qualitative data? Qualitative information is placed into categories, such as eye colour. The categories themselves may have characteristics that enable the researcher to gain insight into the data. One insight is the ordering of the categories. Qualitative data variables may be 'nominal', when they are assigned a category with no natural ordering (see Fig. 4.1). Sex is an example taking the named categories male and female. There is no objective way to place one category 'higher', 'larger', 'better', or 'clearer' than the other category. 'Ordinal' variables have categories that have a natural or objective order (see Fig. 4.1). For example, the categories of pain that a patient reports are ordinal: absent, mild, moderate or severe. These represent increasing severity of pain, whilst maintaining the qualitative, subjective assessment of the pain experience.

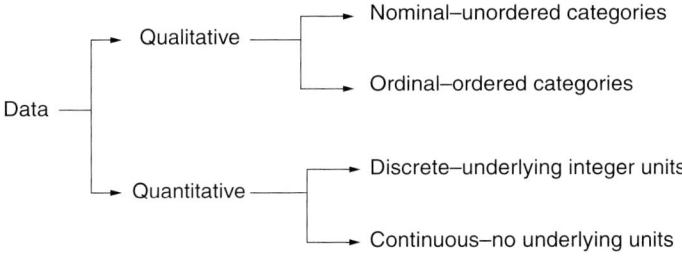

Fig. 4.1. Data types.

A commonly used method for collecting subjective data is to use the Likert type scale (most properly pronounced 'Lick - Urt'). The Likert scale, invented by American psychologist Rensis Likert in the 1930s, places a person's level of agreement or disagreement with a statement using a five-point scale. A respondent could be given a statement such as 'Football is a great sport' and asked their opinion from one of the following five reactions: strongly disagree, disagree, neither agree nor disagree, agree, strongly agree. The data collected is qualitative, but it is placed into a natural order and therefore Likert scales are ordinal data.

Quantitative data may be continuous or discrete

Numerical variables may also be classified into two types: discrete or continuous (see Fig. 4.1). The distinction is less clear sometimes, and there may be disagreement in this distinction. A discrete variable takes whole numerical values, such as –1, 0, 1, 2 and 3. The number of hospital episodes that a patient has experienced is a good example of a discrete variable. Continuous variables have no such limitation on values. Weight can be 87.2345678 kg and there is no restriction to the precision. Note however that continuous variables are not usually collected with such fine detail. It is possible that the weight will be recorded as 87 kg, but weight is still a continuous variable even though it may only be recorded in a whole number of kilograms. A similar example is age where the age last birthday, in years, is recorded.

Defining scales for data

With quantitative data, there are two forms of scale. The 'ratio scale' is where the data have equidistant values and it includes a zero value. For example, height is a ratio scale as 0 kg is possible where multiplication and division are also possible. So for example a person weighing 100 kg is twice the weight of someone weighing 50 kg. A person weighing 70 kg is 10 kg more than a person weighing 60 kg, whilst a person weighing 80 kg is also 10 kg more than someone weighing 70 kg.

There is another type of quantitative scale, known as the 'interval scale'. Interval scales, in the same way as ratio scales, have equidistant values, but they do not contain a meaningful zero. For example using the Celsius scale for temperature, 30 degrees Celsius is 10 degrees more than 20 degrees, which is itself 10 degrees more than 10 degrees. However, it is not appropriate to say that 20 degrees is twice as 'hot' as 10 degrees. This is solved by placing temperature onto a ratio scale, where there is a zero value, known as absolute zero, which is equivalent to –273 degrees Celsius.

An important feature of qualitative data is that the intervals between the categories are not defined. The categories may be assigned a 'label' but this does not mean that the information contained in that variable is constructed from that number. This is a common misconception, and is illustrated in Box 4.1.

Summary

Data are collected in epidemiological research and stored as variables. Understanding the types of data that are present in a study determines the statistical analysis and

Box 4.1. Agreeable disagreeableness

Imagine a study in which a student is trying to collect opinions by asking people if they agree or disagree with a statement, using a Likert scale: 'A doctor should treat a prostitute in the same way as an Olympic gold medallist'.

The student labels the values from one to five, and then uses these values to calculate a mean average.

Is it possible to calculate an 'average opinion' in this way? Unfortunately not. By assigning a numerical value to their data, the student makes the assumption that the response to each question relates in proportion to the other possible responses. So, they're assuming that the people who were in the category 'disagree' (category '2') are actually twice as agreeable as people in 'strongly disagree' (category '1'). The statement 'twice as agreeable' is not justifiable with these data – qualitative data should not be combined in this way. It's a common mistake, but there are other, more appropriate ways to handle these data.

presentation of data. The data that are collected may be divided into two broad types: qualitative and quantitative. Qualitative data are based on subjective measurement, and usually stored as categories. The counts of measurements in the categories may give rise to numeric data. Qualitative data may be categorized into ordinal and nominal. Ordinal data are divided into categories with a natural ordering to them, such as used by the Likert scale, whilst in contrast nominal data have no natural ordering, such as eye colour.

Quantitative data, collected as numbers, may be divided into discrete and continuous data. The division is based on whether the distribution of the underlying data is continuous, or is based on single, whole, discrete numbers. The scale used by the quantitative data is important, as a ratio scale allows multiplication and division of the data as it contains a true zero. Interval scale quantitative data still allows the comparison of differences between data, but they cannot be divided or multiplied in any sensible way.

Self-test questions

Q 4.1.1: Name the four main types of data.

Q 4.1.2: Assign each of these sets of data to a type, qualitative nominal, qualitative ordinal, quantitative discrete, quantitative continuous:
A Height
B Sex
C Number of children
D Type of degree (BA, BSc, MBChB)
E Marital status
F Cancer staging (I, II, III, IV)

Q 4.1.3: For these sets of data, determine the scale (ratio scale, or interval scale):
A Weight
B Number of moles on a person's skin

C Date of a person's birthday

D Altitude above sea-level

E Income in dollars

4.2 Presenting Data

- Pre-requisite sections: 4.1.
- Learning outcome: By the end of the section you should be able to summarize data in a table and graphically.

All research produces data, and medical research is no different; an epidemiologist produces mountains of data. One of their jobs is to summarize and present data for other epidemiologists, statisticians, clinicians, politicians and the public to understand. Data presentation justifies your inferences, influences people and allows you to present cogent arguments.

Over the years, data presentation has formed a core tool in the success of epidemiology. John Snow used simple mapping to work out the source of the cholera outbreak and Florence Nightingale helped to develop, and then used to great effect, a presentation tool known as the polar area diagram. In 1858 she published data on sanitation in India which made an enormous impact on soldiers' lives, such that over the next 15 years mortality had reduced from 69 per 1000 to 18 per 1000. Despite their simplicity, visual presentations of epidemiological data have influenced public health practice and policy around the world.

A good starting point is the frequency table

A 'frequency table' records the distribution of the data as a description of the manner in which values of a variable are scattered, or placed. The number of times each value, or range of values, occurs is counted up and recorded as a frequency. The percentage of values gives the relative frequency.

As a simple example, let's imagine we have a study that wishes to collect two sets of data. The first, which in this case is the independent variable, is the blood group of people. The data for the 16 participants in the study is shown in the left hand part of Fig. 4.2. A frequency table is constructed by counting the number of participants in each blood group, and recording those within

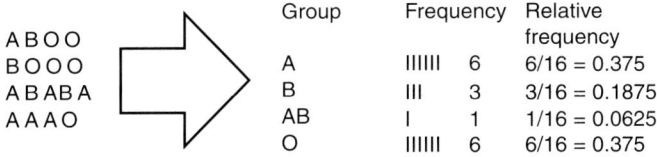

Fig. 4.2. Frequency table from ABO blood group data.

their relevant group. For example there were six people with blood group A, and only one with group AB.

The relative frequency is then calculated by dividing the number in the group by the total number in all groups (see Fig. 4.2). This is the most straightforward approach to displaying and summarizing the data for a nominal, ordinal, or even for a discrete quantitative variable. When a quantitative variable, particularly a continuous variable, is displayed in a frequency table a range of values is used for each category in the table. The person constructing the table may use pre-defined ranges, such as pre-existing categories used by other people in the same field, or they create their own ranges for the table.

Display data in categories as bar charts or pie charts

A simple method for displaying frequency data is the bar chart. Bar charts are appropriate for qualitative and quantitative discrete variables. A 'bar' is drawn for each category with its length proportional to the frequency in that category. The bars are separated by small gaps to indicate that the variable is categorical or discrete. Please note the labels for the axes, and that each bar has the same width. Figure 4.3 displays the blood group data as a bar chart.

Pie charts display categorical and quantitative data

Pie charts are used for categorical variables, and may be used for numeric data, although this is rare. A circular 'pie' is split into sections with the area of each section proportional to the frequency of the corresponding category. Figure 4.4 shows the same data as the bar chart in Fig. 4.3.

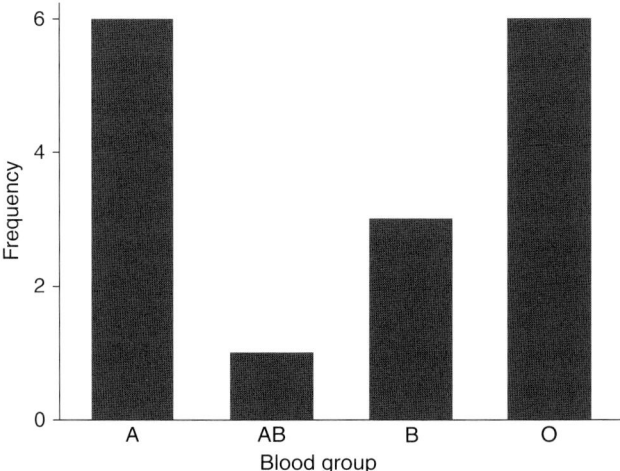

Fig. 4.3. Bar chart of frequency of ABO blood group data.

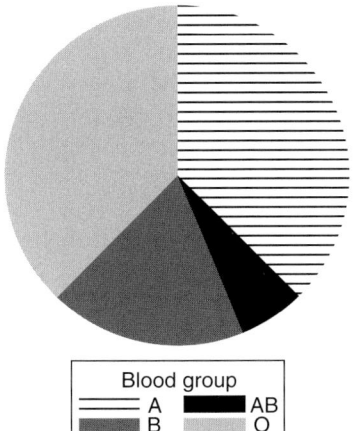

Blood group
A | AB
B | O

Fig. 4.4. Pie chart of frequency of ABO blood group data.

Histograms display quantitative data

It is slightly less straightforward to display data that does not form natural groups. The ABO blood group data has clear groups. What about a variable such as age? You may argue that the number of years is a natural break, and this may be true. But we must remember that this break remains artificial. It is also often too fine for sensible presentation of data and the analyst may wish to expand the group size.

Age will probably be recorded as a number of days, or months, or years. Most people may report their date of birth, which has the resolution of one day. The construction of a frequency table may use pre-defined ranges, such as 0–4, 5–9, 10–14 years. Or the analyst may choose other categories, which may be driven by the data itself.

Histograms are an appropriate way to display visually the frequency distribution of continuous or discrete variables. The first step in producing a histogram is to split the variable's range into 'classes', or 'bins'. Note that sometimes classes will be chosen with different widths, especially when there are fewer observations in part of the range. The classes are used to group the values of the variable so that a frequency table can be composed.

A histogram is then drawn similar to a bar chart but with no gap between the bars. It is very important to note that the area of the bar, rather than just its height, is proportional to the frequency. Consequently, the height is proportional to the frequency divided by the class width. In practice, when using software to produce a histogram, the 'bin' widths are assigned to be equal. As an example, Box 4.2 shows birth weight data, in kg for a survey you have conducted.

Box 4.2. Birth weight data in kg

2.35, 2.28, 3.05, 4.5, 2.55, 2.31, 2.19, 3.59, 2.96, 3.46, 3.48, 2.4, 3.05, 3.48, 2.96, 2.61, 2.24, 2.83, 2.97, 3.02, 5.10

With no prior empirical reason for using other categories, we choose to use a bin of width 1 kg. This makes the interpretation straightforward. Figure 4.5 shows two histograms of the birth weight data with a bin width of 1kg. The two histograms demonstrate how simple and straightforward changes to the way the histogram is constructed can lead to differences in interpretation. Figure 4.5a has a starting point for the bins of 2 kg, and Fig. 4.5b has a starting point of 1.5 kg.

Boxplots or box-and-whisker plots avoid using the mean

One nice graphical summary of data distributions for quantitative data is a boxplot, also known as a box-and-whisker plot. Figure 4.6 shows a boxplot for the birth weight data. The 'box' covers the inter-quartile range, which is a measure of the spread of the data. The box contains a central line which represents the average

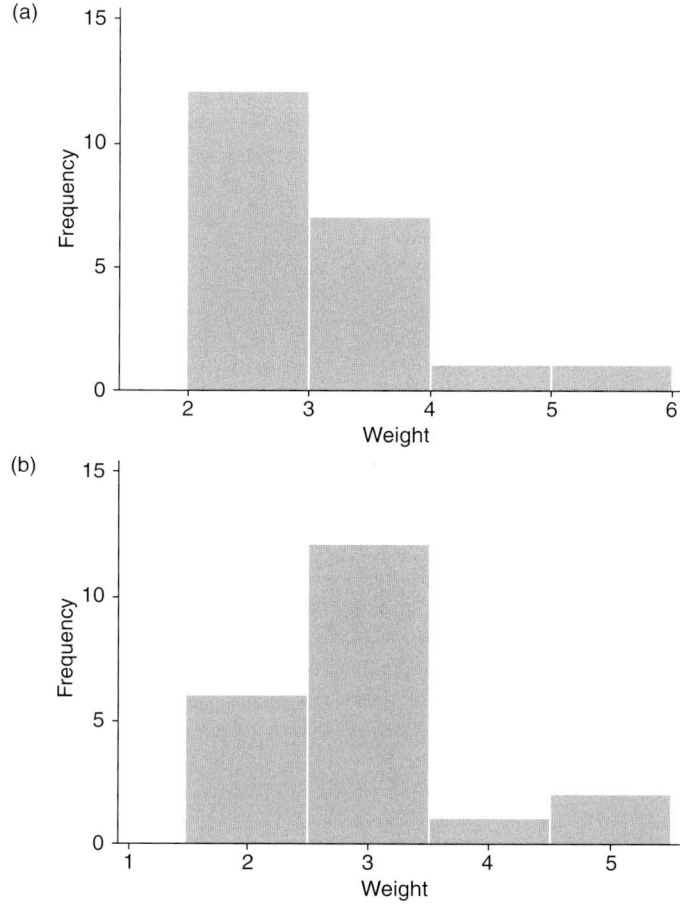

Fig. 4.5. (a) Histogram of birth weight data, starting point 2 kg. (b) Histogram of birth weight data, starting point 1.5kg.

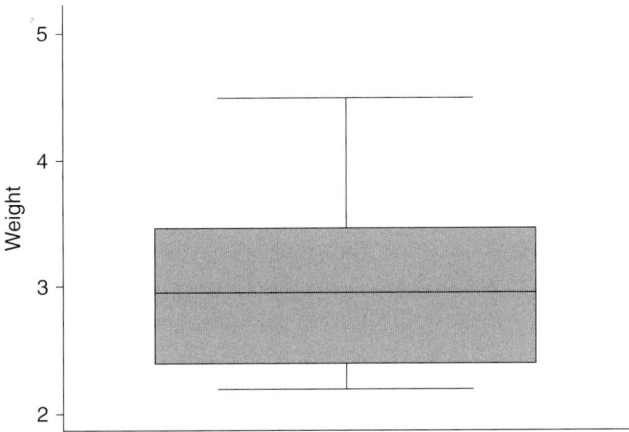

Fig. 4.6. Boxplot of the ABO blood group data.

measured by the median. The 'whiskers' extend to cover the rest of the range of the data. These are introduced in Sections 4.3 and 4.4.

A possible outlier in our data has been identified and is shown, which is a baby with a large birth weight. The identification of outliers is important. In fact there are no real outliers in the birth weight data, but the most extreme value should be checked for data entry or recording errors. It is possible to make typing errors such as writing 29.6 rather than 2.96 kg.

Scatterplots display two sets of data

So far we have looked at displaying a single set of data using bar charts, pie charts and boxplots. It is usual for a research project to have more than one variable, and the researchers will often want to know how these data relate to each other. We may use a scatterplot to examine the association between two quantitative variables, which may be either discrete or continuous.

Taking the birth weight example further, imagine we have a gestational age for each baby born. This means that the data is 'paired' in that there are two measurements, one birth weight and the other gestational age, for each baby. These data are displayed in Fig. 4.7. The horizontal axis, known as the x-axis, is used to show the 'independent' variable, that it is not affected by the other measurement. In this case the gestational age is the independent variable, and the birth weight is the dependent variable which is displayed on the vertical axis, or y-axis.

The importance of displaying data graphically

In 1973 a statistician (Anscombe, 1973) produced four data sets with exactly the same statistical properties, yet which when inspected graphically illustrate the

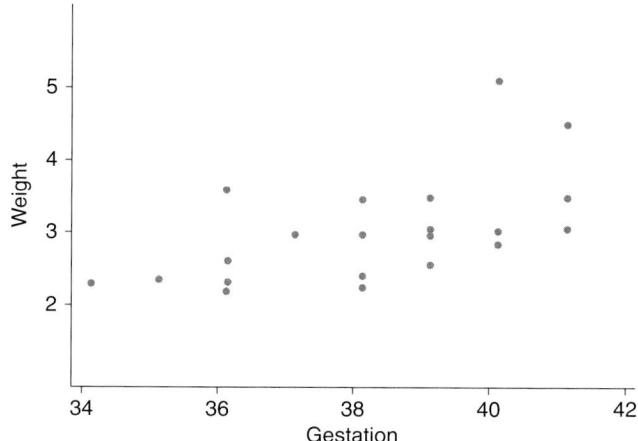

Fig. 4.7. Scatterplot of birth weight and gestational age.

importance of displaying data. Each data set consists of 11 pairs of data points, and was constructed so that each set of data has the same mean and spread, correlation and linear regression line. However, when these data are displayed they are clearly very different (see Fig. 4.8). In this vein, it's essential to use data presentation in statistical work, particularly when looking at data for the first time. There is an adage that essentially says people use statistics in the same way a drunk uses a lamppost: more for support than illumination. Avoid diving straight into summarizing the numbers and see what comes from displaying data visually. It often adds an illumination that is not present with numerical summaries of data.

Summary

Epidemiologists are able to summarize and present their data using a variety of methods. A frequency table displays the number of times each value is counted. These can be displayed using simple methods such as using a scatterplot, boxplot or histogram. How data is displayed can have a significant impact on the message derived from the data.

Self-test questions

Q 4.2.1: For each of these studies, decide which graphical methods should be used to display the data collected:
A Ethnic group of people in a supermarket
B The marks, out of 100, students in a class received for an assessment
C Number of moles counted for a group of teenagers
D Lengths of children at birth
E Lengths of children at birth and their gestational age

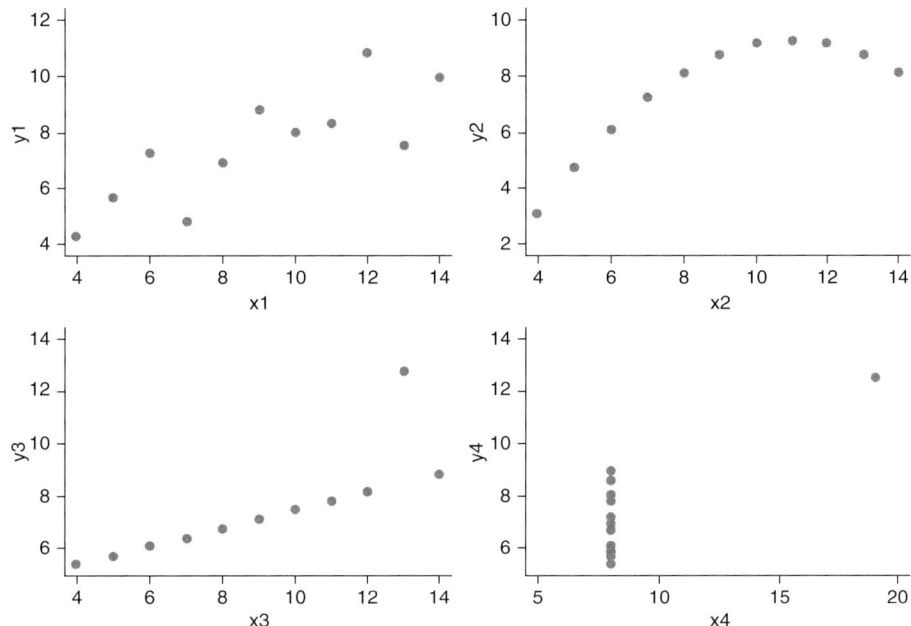

Fig. 4.8. Anscombe's quartet.

Q 4.2.2: True or false? The independent variable is usually displayed on the horizontal (x) axis when constructing a scatterplot.

Q 4.2.3: A boxplot displays which of these summaries of data?
A Mean
B Median
C Mode
D Standard deviation
E Inter-quartile range
F Outliers

4.3 Measures of Location

- Pre-requisite sections: 4.1, 4.2.
- Learning outcome: By the end of this section you should be able to describe measures of location and their meaning.

When data is collected, the first thing you may ask is what is the 'normal', 'typical' or 'average' value of the measurements that you have made? The epidemiologist may use data to answer this question, by calculating a measure of location. This fits with a statistical approach to the data; it is common for data to have a 'central tendency', that is data in some way clusters around a central measure. It is the researcher's role to determine and calculate the most appropriate measure of central tendency.

The average measure is partly determined by the data type

The data type should be taken into account when determining the measure of location that is most appropriate. One of the most commonly used measures of location is the 'mean'. This is most appropriate for quantitative data that has a central tendency. The mean of a sample is calculated by summing all the values and dividing by the total number of values. In mathematical terms, we refer to the number of values as n, and the sample values are described as x_1, x_2 up to x_n. Writing this as an equation, the sample mean is given by:

$$\bar{x} = \frac{\sum_{i=1}^{n} x_i}{n}$$

where the subscript i indicates that all values of x from 1 to n should be used; this is known as indexing. The Greek letter Σ, known as sigma, indicates the sum of the values: the analyst must add up all values of x. The 'bar', or line, over x is a convention indicating that this is the 'mean of x'. This is also, more specifically, known as an arithmetic mean.

Weighted means are used to adjust the average

A modification of the usual arithmetic mean is a weighted mean. Again in symbols, the weighted mean is:

$$\bar{x}' = \sum_{i=1}^{n} w_i x_i$$

where w_i is the weight you wish to give for each value of x_i. The w_i should add up to one. As an example, imagine an assessment with two marks, where you received 50% in the first test, and 70% in the second test. If these tests were equally weighted then the arithmetic mean would be:

$$\bar{x} = \frac{50 + 70}{2} = 60$$

Therefore you would receive an overall mark of 60%. This may be rewritten as where the multiplier of 0.5 represents the fact that each test is weighted equally, one half of the overall value for each test. And therefore the weighted mean, where each mark is equally weighted is:

$$\bar{x} = (50 \times 0.5) + (70 \times 0.5) = 60$$

Now imagine that the first test was more important in the tutor's mind than the second and they wished to reflect this in the overall mark. The tutor might decide that the first test is worth 60% of the overall mark. The new average will be:

$$\bar{x}' = (50 \times 0.6) + (70 \times 0.4) = 58$$

You would receive 58% in the assessment.

The normal distribution or bell-shaped curve

The normal distribution, also known as the Gaussian distribution or bell-curve, is a statistical distribution that is widely used in epidemiology. The equation for generating the values is:

$$f(x) = \frac{1}{\sqrt{2\pi \times SD^2}} \, e^{-\frac{(x-\bar{x})^2}{2 \times SD^2}}$$

where SD is the standard deviation, $\bar{x}$ the mean, x are the sample values of data, e is the exponent of the value, and π is the value of pi. You really do not need to be overly concerned with this equation, all statistical packages will calculate these where you need them.

When you calculate this distribution it forms a curve, such as the one shown in Fig. 4.9 with a mean of zero and a standard deviation of one. It has some important features, one of which is that the curve is symmetric around the mean value.

Median is the middle value

Another measure of location, or average, is the median. This is the value below which half of the distribution lies, also known as the 50th percentile. In a sample with an odd number of samples, that is n is an odd number, the median is the middle value of the sorted sample. If there is an even number of samples, n is even, then the median is a value midway between the middle two values. The median of the two test marks, 50% and 70%, is 60%.

The median is useful for data types where the mean is not appropriate. For example, a Likert scale is a five-point scale in response to a question. The scale allows a response of strongly disagree through to strongly agree. It is tempting for the analyst

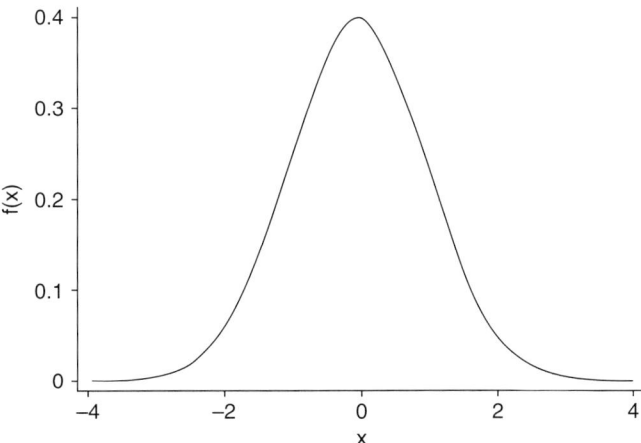

Fig. 4.9. Normal distribution.

to assign a value to each of the categories, for example 1, 2, 3, 4 and 5, and to use the mean to estimate the location of the responses. This is wholly inappropriate as we cannot justify that a person in category 2 for example, who disagreed, is actually twice as agreeable or disagreeable as people in category 1, who strongly disagreed. Under these circumstances the median is an appropriate measure of location.

Mode is the most frequent value

A third measure of location is the mode, which is defined as the most frequently occurring value in a data set. If we are interested in the number that occurs most often from those listed here, 1, 2, 2, 3, 5, 7, 7, 7, 8, 10, then the mode is 7, as that occurs the most often.

To determine the mode, you need to order the scores as shown above, and then count each one. In some distributions there is more than one mode value, such as one with two peaks in the data known as a bi-modal distribution. If the distribution is truly normal, the mean, median and mode are all equal to each other. The mode is not often used, partly because it may only be used where there are discrete values. It is probably most often useful with the nominal data type.

Extreme values are known as outliers

Extreme values are unusually large or small values of a variable we are interested in. The definition of 'extreme' is dependent on the situation, for example it may be a value (or range of values) that could occur 1 in 50 times, 1 in 1000 or 1 in 10,000 times. It may be a very high value or a very low value, but it must be a value whose occurrence is rare. A good example is abnormally high weight in children (Kwon *et al.*, 2006). Statistical analysis of these extreme values aims to examine their occurrence to make best use of the data. As with all other areas of epidemiology we want to understand the processes generating these extremes and if possible predict any future values.

It is up to the epidemiologist to decide what will be considered abnormal and this is usually done using a consensus method. All outliers should be investigated carefully as often they contain valuable information about the process under investigation. Also outliers can shed light on the data gathering and recording processes.

A naive approach to dealing with outliers is to delete them from the data. Before considering the elimination of outliers from the data, ask the question 'why did they appear?' and whether it is likely similar values will continue to appear. If an outlier is a genuine result, it is important. The outlier might show an extreme form of behaviour under study.

The average may be affected by outliers

Imagine a set of data where there is an outlier. Using the mean to estimate the location of the data will result in the outlier being summed with the rest of the data, and therefore the mean will be closer to the outlying value than if the outlier were excluded. The median will not be affected in this way, as the median will not change with an outlier added to the data.

Summary

Measures of location are the often first step in our analysis of data. There are three simple measures of location: the mean, median and mode. The type of measure of location is partly dependent upon the data type, and the occurrence of outliers.

The usual measure of central tendency is known as the 'average'. The lay public, and the media, use the term 'average' in many different contexts. It is often used in a derogatory way to indicate something of poor quality, as illustrated in Box 4.3. In statistics it has a specific meaning, and relates to the 'central' point or measure of the distribution of measurements.

Self-test questions

Q 4.3.1: What is the mean, median and mode of these data?
2.2, 4.4, 6.6, 1.1, 7.7, 15.15, 5.5, 3.3

Q 4.3.2: What is the outlier in Q 4.3.1? What is the impact of the outlier in Q 4.3.1?

Q 4.3.3: The average for the normal distribution is:
A Mean
B Median
C Mode

Q 4.3.4: True or False? The mean is affected by outliers.

Q 4.3.5: The median is based on which percentile?
A 0
B 25
C 50
D 75
E 100

Box 4.3. Half of all doctors are worse than average

A student reading a newspaper headline is at first alarmed at what it seems to say about the state of the health system: 'Half of all doctors are worse than average'.

Looking a little closer at the article, it turns out the statistic was taken from a questionnaire given to patients asking them to rate their doctor's diagnosis and treatment, and the journalist had then calculated the median average. To calculate the median, you find the point in the data where half of the observations lie below and half lie above the median value. So, by definition, half of all the doctors evaluated are below this average. The headline implying that half of all doctors were found to be below standard by their patients is therefore not to be taken at face value!

4.4 Measures of Spread

- Pre-requisite sections: 4.1–4.3.
- Learning outcome: By the end of this section you should be able to describe the meaning of measures of spread.

Along with the information about the location of the data, it is important to provide information about the spread of the values around the location. The reason for this requirement may be illustrated with a simple thought experiment. Consider needing to treat a group of people. You have been told that their mean age is 40 years. However, this group could be composed of very different sorts of people. You might have a group that includes children and older people, rather than a group with ages varying from 38 to 42 years. This is an issue of precision, where a set of data that lies close to the location is a precise set of data, and should not be confused with accuracy.

The 'range' of a variable is defined by the smallest and largest value in the sample or the difference between the smallest and largest values. For large samples, however, other measures of spread showing the spread for the majority of individuals are preferred.

Standard deviation is the average of the spread

A second measure of spread, known as the standard deviation (abbreviated here to 'SD'), is widely used and should be used in conjunction with the mean as the measure of location. The SD is calculated as the extent the values in the sample vary from its mean. When the values are tightly bunched together, the SD is small. When the values are spread widely you have a relatively large SD. The SD is only appropriate for quantitative data.

We can loosely interpret the SD as a measure of the average distance of all of the data values from the mean. In symbols this is

$$SD = \sqrt{\frac{\sum_{i=1}^{n}(x_i - \overline{x})^2}{n-1}}$$

To calculate the sample SD follow these steps:

1. Calculate the mean.
2. Subtract the mean from every value.
3. Square each of the values obtained in step 2. Add these squared values together to give the sum of the squares value.
4. Divide the final result obtained from step 3 by the total number of values in the sample minus 1. This is known as the variance.
5. Take the square root of the result obtained in step 4. This is the SD.

As an example, the number of births each week in a particular village were recorded as 4, 3, 7, 2, 4. To calculate the SD:

1. The mean number of births is given by

$$\frac{4+3+7+2+5}{5} = 4 \; births \, per \, week$$

2. Subtracting the mean from each value gives 0, –1, 3, –2, 0
3. Squaring and adding these gives $(0 + 1 + 9 + 4 + 0) = 14$
4. Dividing by the number of weeks less one gives $14/4 = 3.5$
5. The SD is the square root of 3.5, which is 1.87 births per week.

The standard deviation compares proportions of the sample to the mean

The SD may now be used to infer the proportion of the sample that lies at different distances from the mean. For example:

- One SD away from the mean in either direction, greater or lesser, accounts for somewhere around 68% of the values in the group.
- Two SDs away from the mean accounts for roughly 95% of the values.
- Three SDs accounts for about 99% of the sample.

Why is this useful? The standard deviation will determine how diverse the values in your sample are. This is explored in Box 4.4, in the context of a court case. A statistician may use the central 95% of their sample to represent the range in which they place some confidence.

Take an example where you are comparing calorie intake for different schools. Let's say Springfield Primary School has a higher mean test score than Leeds Primary School. Your first reaction might be to say that the children at Springfield are eating more. But a larger standard deviation for one school tells you that there are relatively more kids at that school scoring toward one extreme or the other. By asking a few follow-up questions you might find Springfield's mean was skewed because the school district sends all of the poorer children to Springfield, or that Leeds' scores were reduced because students have recently been given nutrition classes.

The standard deviation has one undesirable aspect. Given it is based on the mean, one or two extreme scores easily influence the standard deviation in the same way the mean may also be affected. Atypical scores in a distribution, known as outliers, can affect the distribution's SD.

Inter-quartile range is used with the median

Recall that the median is the value for which 50% of the data in a sample have values which are less. We will now define a measure of spread that can be used with the median. The lower quartile, often called Q1, is defined as that value for which 25% of individuals have values that are less. Similarly the upper quartile, Q3, is the value for which 75% of individuals have values that are less. This means that the lower quartile, median and upper quartile divide the distribution into quarters.

There is no universal agreement on choosing the quartile values. One rule, which we use here, is to first use the median to divide the ordered data set into two halves. When calculating Q1 and Q3, do not include the median value into the halves. The lower quartile value is the median of the lower half of the data. The upper quartile value is the median of the upper half of the data.

In the following scenario, a professor of statistics is acting as an expert witness for a doctor who is being sued. The plaintiff has based their case on a single study, the reliability of which the professor calls into question. She is now defending her position to the lawyers for the plaintiff…

Lawyer: Professor, can you tell us the problems you have with the study that my client says proves the defendant wrong?

Professor: The study the plaintiff is referring to is too small.

Lawyer: Can you explain to the court what you mean by this?

Professor: There are many reasons why a study might not be good enough to answer a question. The simplest is the number of people in the study. A study that is too small will not be sufficient.

Lawyer: How do you know when a study is big enough?

Professor: This is a difficult question. Do you know about the Paradox of Sorites? This paradox starts with 1,000,000 grains of sand. The question is posed: is this a heap of sand?

Lawyer: Yes, of course.

Professor: We now remove a grain of sand. Is it still a heap of sand?

Lawyer: Yes.

Professor: Ok, so we continue removing grains of sand. There are two premises here: one, that 1,000,000 grains of sand is a heap of sand, and two: that a heap of sand minus one grain is still a heap. Taking this to its logical conclusion, one grain of sand, or even no grains of sand, remains a heap. If it is no longer a heap, when did it stop being one? This is the same for people in a study: when is a study too small for it to be meaningful? It's a paradox as there is no true answer. But statisticians have defined, for many years, a cut-off value of 5%, for achieving statistical significance.

Lawyer: 5% of what?

Professor: The researcher can perform tests of probability on the study and come up with the probability that, under the null hypothesis, the result occurs. The researchers discovered that, were this hypothesis not true, the probability of this result occurring by chance was less than 5%.

Lawyer: So we can say this study is false?

Professor: We need to be more circumspect. We can say that, based on this study, there is not sufficient evidence.

The inter-quartile range (IQR) is Q1 to Q3. Between these two values, half of the distribution lies. Note that this can be used as a measure of spread for continuous and discrete metric variables and also for ordered variables. For example if we have data: 1, 2, 3, 4, 5, the Q1 is 1.5, Q3 is 4.5 (as the median value 3 is excluded) and the IQR is 1.5 to 4.5. If we have data: 7, 15, 36, 39, 40, 41, the Q1 is 15, and Q3 is 40 and the IQR is 15 to 40. This is because we do not exclude the median value.

As an aside, the term quartile is similar to other '…tile' words, and you should be careful to use these in an appropriate way. The quartile is not the set of values, that is a quarter, the quartile is the divide between two quarters. Similarly, quintiles divide fifths and tertiles divide thirds.

Boxplot displays median and quartiles

A boxplot is a graphical representation of five numbers: the smallest value (the 0th percentile), the lower quartile (Q1; the 25th percentile), the median (the 50th percentile), the upper quartile (Q3; the 75th percentile), and the largest value (the 100th percentile). Boxplots are useful for having a quick visual idea of the distribution of a data set. Referring to the birth weight data, Fig. 4.6 shows a boxplot. The Q1 is 2.4 kg and Q3 3.46 kg. These are shown as the bottom and top boundaries of the box.

Summary

By using measures of spread, such as the range, standard deviation or inter-quartile range, we can start to develop a level of confidence in our predictions about our data. Measures of spread are the second step in our analysis of data after calculating the location of the data.

Self-test questions

Q 4.4.1: What are the measures of spread?

Q 4.4.2: What are the measures of spread for these data?
2.2, 4.4, 6.6, 1.1, 7.7, 15.15, 5.5, 3.3

Q 4.4.3: What is the impact of the outlier on the measures of spread?

Q 4.4.4: The lower quartile:
A Contains the top 25% of the data.
B Contains the lower 25% of the data.
C Divides the two halves of the data.
D Divides the lower 25% from the upper 75% of the data.

4.5 Prevalence of Disease

- Pre-requisite sections: 1.4, 1.5, 3.4.
- Learning outcome: By the end of the section you should be able to define the meaning of prevalence and describe the way prevalence is used in epidemiology.

Prevalence, or point prevalence, is the proportion of individuals in a population that have a particular outcome at a particular time. The measure of prevalence is used to define and describe the burden of a disease, and it helps researchers, physicians or other health professionals. It can be used by epidemiologists, healthcare providers, government agencies and insurers to assist in their work.

When we define prevalence we usually mean 'extent', but in the scientific community we are generally meaning 'proportion'. This is expressed as a percentage and is different from incidence. Prevalence is the measurement of all individuals with a disease within a particular period of time. Incidence is the measurement of the number of individuals who newly contract a disease during a period of time.

Prevalence is useful for service planning and cause

There are two main reasons that we need to know the amount of disease in a population. The first is to inform service provision. Knowledge about the amount of disease is used to inform decision making for health service resources and for public health. The second is to compare the amount observed with another time (for example before and after an intervention), or another place (for example the north and the south hemispheres of the globe), or another group of persons (males with females for example). These characteristics of time, place and person are often referred to as the 'epidemiological triad'. If differences exist between these, then something may be learned about the disease, and risk factors may be identified.

Prevalence is the proportion of the population with disease

Box 4.5 introduces the bath analogy, a useful concept for working through the impact of changes on incidence and prevalence, and it is expanded on in Box 4.6. The prevalence of a disease at that particular time, in that place, is the number of people with the outcome, those in the bathtub, compared to all of those in the population, both with and without the outcome. In symbols:

$$P = \frac{n_1}{n}$$

where n_1 is the number of individuals in the population with the disease, and n is the number of individuals in the population at risk of developing the disease, including individuals with

---

Box 4.5. Introducing the bath analogy

Prevalence is used to measure the amount, or volume, of disease in a population. It is different to the term 'incidence', but both terms are sometimes used interchangeably in lay language, particularly in the media. A useful analogy for understanding these terms is to imagine a bathtub:

The water in the tub represents the total number of cases of disease in the population: this is the prevalent pool of cases. What may now happen? The plug may be taken out. This represents people being cured, dying, or moving away.

---

the disease. Further exploration of prevalence can be done by expressing it for subgroups of the population based on different denominator data such as age or gender.

As an example, a GP wishes to find out the number of people with asthma in their population. The researcher has determined the time point for the survey and the method for observing the number of people with and without asthma. The researcher discovered that in their practice population of 4876, there were 190 people with a record of symptoms of asthma in their medical records at that time. Therefore, the prevalence of asthma in the practice was:

$$P = \frac{190}{4876} = 0.039$$

which represents 3.9 persons having asthma per 100 at that point in time.

Prevalence may be measured at a point, period or lifetime

In epidemiology, point prevalence is a measure of the proportion of people in a population who have a disease or condition at a particular time, like a snap shot of the disease in time. This is in contrast to period prevalence which is a measure of the proportion of people in a population who have a disease or condition over a specific period of time, say a season, or a year. Lifetime prevalence is the number of individuals in a population that at some point in their life, up to the time of assessment, have experienced a disease. The total number of people who have experienced an outcome during their lifetime is compared to the total number of individuals. In the same way as for point and period prevalence, the lifetime prevalence is expressed as a proportion.

Note that common diseases with short duration, such as influenza, will have low point prevalence, because when a person is cured they are no longer a prevalent case. Using the analogy the cases are removed through the plughole. Diseases with a long duration such as rheumatoid arthritis or diabetes will have high prevalence, especially when the disease does not give a higher mortality rate. The prevalence of a disease will increase when the number of cases increases. Cases for a disease that is incurable, such as HIV or diabetes, will increase with new incident cases.

Incidence, cure, migration and death all change prevalence

The prevalence of a disease in a population will change over time. New cases are added to the pool of cases, with each new diagnosis, known as incident cases. Cases will remain within the prevalent pool until either that person is cured of the disease, or they die or migrate out of the population. The bath analogy extends further, with each new drip from the tap considered a new case. The quicker the tap drips, the quicker the prevalent pool may increase. To balance this, cases of disease will leave the pool, which is analogous to the water leaving the bathtub. If a cure is possible, patients that were once cases may re-join the population at risk. When cure actually gives lifelong immunity, the cured people do not rejoin the population at risk.

For example, imagine a new disease that takes a long time to develop symptoms and has been able to spread widely in a community, and a preventive measure has been introduced. Despite this, the prevalence will remain high even though incidence is low. This means there are many existing cases, but not many new ones. HIV is a good example of this progression.

Conversely, a disease that is easily transmitted but has a short duration between transmission and when symptoms first present might spread widely but is likely to have a low prevalence at any given point (due to its short duration). Incidence is more useful when describing diseases of short duration, such as chickenpox.

Examples of using prevalence

A team at the Office for National Statistics wishes to know how well general practices are progressing in meeting some of the targets set out in their National Service Framework for coronary heart disease. Researchers use data from primary care databases such as the General Practice Research Database to examine what proportion of patients with conditions such as arterial fibrillation and heart failure are receiving appropriate treatments. As the data are longitudinal, researchers are able to examine time trends in treatment rates. The large size of the database also allows them to look to see how treatment rates vary in different age groups and between genders. Finally they use the information on age-sex prevalence rates with population projections to predict the likely change in the number of cases in future years. They find that because of the ageing of the population, the number of people suffering from conditions such as arterial fibrillation that are most common in the elderly will increase substantially in future years. This in turn will have important implications for stroke services and anticoagulation clinics.

Summary

The prevalence of a disease is used to measure the volume of that disease in the population. We introduced a bath analogy to explain the way prevalence can be measured, and how it changes with incidence, cure, migration and mortality.

Self-test questions

Q 4.5.1: Which one, or more, of the following may affect the prevalence of a disease in a population?
A Inwards migration
B Outwards migration
C Deaths
D Births
E Treatment
F Cure

Q 4.5.2: In a GP population with 4134 patients, 2467 of whom are female, the clinical information system showed that 47 had cervical cancer, and a further 7 had been diagnosed with it but had been cured. Calculate the point prevalence of cervical cancer.

Q 4.5.3: In a city, a disease is suddenly curable. Does the prevalence:
A Increase?
B Decrease?
C Stay the same?

4.6 Incidence of Disease

- Pre-requisite sections: 1.4, 3.5, 4.5.
- Learning outcome: By the end of this section you should be able to define incidence of disease and how it may be standardized.

The incidence, or more correctly, incidence rate, of an outcome is the extent or rate of occurrence of the outcome. For disease, it specifically refers to the number of new cases of that disease in a population over a period of time, and is expressed as a rate. The bath analogy is explored further in Box 4.6, providing a way to remember the difference between incidence and prevalence.

The epidemiologist must define the population at risk, as a count of the total people that might feasibly develop the outcome. The number at risk may be defined over a time period of, say, 1 year which would give an annual incidence rate. It may be that the population is monitored for a number of years, or for periods shorter than a year.

Count the people in the population at risk

The most straightforward way to measure the underlying population is to use an estimate of the population size at one point in time. For example, the population could be enumerated at the mid-point of the study period. Such a calculation is sufficient if the number of people at risk is reasonably constant over the period of time, and for a large population as the number should not fluctuate significantly.

The number at risk can, however, vary over time and lead to inaccuracies in the estimates. For example, people in a population at risk can be born or die, be recruited into or leave a study at different times, or get the disease under investigation and therefore no longer be part of the population at risk as they have the disease. A study may also need to restrict the case groups. For example, a study interested in the risk of childhood cancer may exclude children born with genetic conditions that predispose to cancer, and these must be excluded from the population at risk.

Box 4.6. Extending the bath analogy

Let's extend the bath analogy from Box 4.5 to illustrate the term 'incidence'. Incidence is the occurrence specifically of new cases, sometimes called 'incidence cases'. In the bath analogy, the tap represents the incidence: the dripping tap adds new cases to the prevalent pool. This can be added to the plughole, which represents the loss of cases from the population through migration, cure or death, to complete the analogy.

The person-years of population at risk must be calculated

In epidemiology, it is common to determine the number of person-years in an underlying population, which then is used to calculate the rate of incidence in relation to person-years. For example, if there is one person in the population and this person is monitored for 10 years, they contribute 10 person-years to the population. If you have 10 people that you monitored for 1 year, they also contribute 10 person-years.

As an example, let us consider a study where office workers, given a new type of chair, are followed to see at what rate they develop lower-back pain, which is the outcome of interest. Not all of the office workers use the new chair for the same length of time: there are differences when the chairs are delivered; some workers do not get on with the chair and stop using it; some workers leave the job and stop using the chair. The study recruits 507 office workers and aims to follow them for 26 weeks. The first person recruited to the study uses the chair for 24 weeks, the next for 3 weeks, and the next for 26 weeks, etc. Adding the number of weeks that each person uses the chair produces a total number of 9876 person-weeks.

Incidence is reported per person per unit time

The incidence rate is the number of new cases, often referred to as the numerator as it is on the top of the equation for calculating incidence, occurring in the pre-defined period divided by the number of people at risk in the population during that same period, known as the denominator. In symbols, the crude incidence rate is:

$$I = \frac{o_t}{n_t}$$

where o_t is the number of observed new cases in the time period t, and n_t is the number of people at risk in the population over the same time period. The resulting number must then be reported per number of persons and per time unit.

Returning to our example in the office it was found that nine people get lower-back pain. The incidence rate of lower-back pain is therefore:

$$I = \frac{9}{9876} = 0.00091$$

This is interpreted as 0.0009 cases per person-week. To obtain a more useful measure, we may wish to calculate the number of new cases per person-year. This is simply obtained by multiplying the incidence rate per week by 52 which gives 0.047, or 47 cases per 1000 person-years (multiply the incidence rate per year by 1000). It is common to express rare outcomes, as is the case for many diseases, in terms of 1000, 10,000, or 100,000 person-years.

Fatality and mortality are different to incidence

Epidemiologists sometimes need to examine the deaths or survival from disease, rather than development of the disease. There are various ways to measure mortality. The case fatality rate from a specific disease is the number of people who die from the disease in a time period divided by the number of people with the disease in that same period. This should be distinguished from the mortality rate of a disease, which is the number of people who die from the disease in the time period divided by the number of people who die in the same period.

Standardizing allows comparisons of incidence between subgroups

An important reason for collecting the incidence of a disease is to help understand the causal factors involved in the aetiology of a disease. One investigation is to compare incidence between geographical areas, between sex groups or between other natural groupings. The crude incidence rate, given above, represents a simple interpretation of the data but is liable to bias when comparing between subgroups or strata. For example, when comparing the incidence rate in two towns, such as Harrogate (with a high average age) and Wakefield (a low average age), the underlying age structure may drive the differences in the incidence rates. If you were interested in non-Hodgkin's lymphoma, which increases in incidence with age, Harrogate would likely have a higher crude incidence rate.

A term you will read and hear about, used a great deal in epidemiology, is 'standardization'. In order for a scientist to compare incidence between, for example different regions, they must first take into account factors which are known to affect the observed incidence. These are known in this situation as strata (singular, stratum). Age is commonly used as an important stratum in determining the rates of disease in a population. For this reason age adjustment is often used to compare underlying incidence rates between two geographical areas. There are two main forms of standardization: 'direct' and 'indirect'.

Directly standardized rates use an external population

The principle underlying directly standardized rates is that the epidemiologist can calculate what would be the observed incidence in a 'standard' population. The directly standardized incidence rate recalculates the crude rate using an external standard population distribution. An important first step is to decide the groups that you wish to define as strata. The strata divide the population into more homogeneous groups based on important characteristics within the population.

The directly standardized rate is calculated as follows:

1. The stratum-specific rates are calculated. A stratum is a subgroup of the individuals in the sample. Two examples are age or sex, classic epidemiology strata.
2. A weighted mean of the stratum-specific rates is taken. The weights are provided by the proportion in each stratum in a standard population.

Let us use a simple, and extreme, example to illustrate this. Imagine there were two adjoining areas with data shown in Table 4.1. The total number of cases of an outcome we are interested in for a single year in each area is 100, with a base population at risk of 5000 people in each area. This amounts to 5000 person-years for each area at risk of the outcome. The crude incidence rate in both Area 1 and Area 2 per 1000 person-years is

Table 4.1. A hypothetical incidence rate example for a single year.

Age group	Area 1			Area 2			Standard population
	Cases	Population	Rate per 1000	Cases	Population	Rate per 1000	
0–4	50	1500	33.33	50	2500	20.00	0.5
5–9	50	3500	14.29	50	2500	20.00	0.5
Total	100	5000	20.00	100	5000	20.00	1
Crude rate			20.00			20.00	
Adjusted rate			23.81			20.00	

$$I = \frac{100}{5000} \times 1000 = 20.00$$

This means that the incidence rate is 20 persons with the disease per 1000 person-years in the population. The data is also divided into two age groups, the strata, and we can see that the proportion in each age group differs between the two areas. If the standard population we are interested in has an equal number of people in each age group in the population then the standard population, which is shown in Table 4.1, would assign equal weightings to 0–4 and 5–9 year olds. In order to calculate the age-adjusted rate we first calculate the stratum-specific rates, in this case the rates for each age group. These are shown in Table 4.1 in the 'Rate per 1000' column. For example the rate specific to 5–9 year olds in Area 1 is:

$$I = \frac{50}{3500} \times 1000 = 14.29$$

The directly standardized rate is an average, using the standard population as weights, of the two stratum-specific rates. In Area 2 the standard population is divided into the two age groups in exactly the same way as the actual population, the age-adjusted rate is exactly the same as the crude rate. However, for Area 1 the adjusted rate per 1000 person-years is:

$$I = (33.33 \times 0.5) + (14.29 \times 0.5) = 23.81$$

From this you can infer that the rates of disease are, if applied to a standard population, higher in Area 1 than in Area 2. This may have relevance for the aetiology of the disease you are examining.

There are many standard populations

The choice of weightings, given by the standard populations, is important and it is common to use an internationally recognized weighting factor. This allows us to represent a realistic standard population and allows a wide range of locations and studies to compare their incidence. Some of the more commonly used weightings are given in Table 4.2. When comparing the incidence rates between subgroups, such as a geographical zone, the researcher must ensure that the same standard population is used.

Table 4.2. Standard populations.

Age group	European	World
0–4	8	8.86
5–9	7	8.69
10–14	7	8.6
15–19	7	8.47
20–24	7	8.22
25–29	7	7.93
30–34	7	7.61
35–39	7	7.15
40–44	7	6.59
45–49	7	6.04
50–54	7	5.37
55–59	6	4.55
60–64	5	3.72
65–69	4	2.96
70–74	3	2.21
75–79	2	1.52
80–84	1	0.91
85+	1	0.63
Total	100	100

Indirectly standardized ratio is used for small numbers

Direct standardization is an important tool for comparing subgroups in epidemiology studies. However, when any one cell contains a small number of cases or even zero cases, such as an older age group in a small area, then directly standardized rates may be biased, and it is more appropriate to use indirect standardization. This may seem confusing as the terms imply that indirect is less powerful than direct but in some circumstances the opposite is true.

Whilst direct standardization offers the incidence for a standard population, indirectly standardized rates are comparing the area to the 'standard incidence rates' for all areas. Indirect standardization may be initially expressed as a ratio of the observed number of cases of the outcome to the expected number applying the overall incidence rates. This generates a standardized incidence ratio, abbreviated to SIR, or when mortality is examined then this is known as the standardized mortality ratio, abbreviated to SMR. The indirectly standardized ratio may then be applied to the overall rates to obtain the indirectly standardized incidence rate.

Let's work through an example using data in Table 4.3, which shows the total number of cases and people in the population at risk for the entire study. There is a calculated incidence rate, per 1 person-year for each of the two age groups. Remember that indirect standardization is used when there are small numbers of cases in any of the groups; this is appropriate for this data.

The individual rates calculated for each age group in the entire data set can be used to apply to the population in Area 1. In this hypothetical example there are only 7 cases in Area 1, and the epidemiologist wishes to see whether there are more or fewer than would be expected for a population of this size.

Table 4.3. A hypothetical example for a standardized incidence ratio (SIR).

Age group	Total			Area 1			
	Cases	Population	Rate per 1	Cases	Population	Expected cases	SIR
0–4	100	4000	0.025	3	150	3.75	0.80
5–9	100	6000	0.017	4	350	5.83	0.69
Total	200	10000		7	500	9.58	0.73

In symbols, the expected number of cases in stratum s in area a is:

$$e_{as} = n_{as} \times I_s$$

where n_{as} is the number of people in the population in stratum s in area a, and I_s is the crude incidence rate for the stratum. So in the example the expected number of cases in Area 1 and the 0–4 year old stratum is:

$$e_{as} = 150 \times 0.025 = 3.75$$

The total number of expected cases is then summed across the stratum-specific expected numbers, which for Area 1 gives 9.58 cases. The standardized incidence ratio is the total number of observed cases divided by the total number of expected cases. In the example we get

$$SIR = \frac{7}{3.75 + 5.83} = 0.73$$

It is also common to see this measure as a percentage, which means the SIR would be reported as 73%, where 100% represents the number of observed cases that you would expect in that area. This tells us that there are 27% fewer cases observed in this area than should be expected applying the whole data set to this area.

The rate is calculated from the ratio

To calculate the indirectly standardized rate for stratum s in area a we apply the overall rate to the ratio for the specific area. So we get:

$$I_{sa} = SIR \times I = 0.73 \times 20.00 = 14.6$$

which shows that the indirectly standardized rate is 14.6 per 1000 person-years.

Cumulative and stratum-specific incidence may offer clues to aetiology

A further step may be taken with the incidence rates, particularly rates using age as a stratum. It is possible to calculate the cumulative incidence of an outcome over a person's lifetime up until a specific age, or for their entire life. This assumes that no other external events affect a person's life. Cumulative incidence is often shown graphically. The cumulative rate is simply calculated by summing the rates for the years prior to the age that you wish to examine.

Stratum-specific incidence rates have been used earlier in this section to create a standardized incidence rate. These measures are potentially useful and interesting in their own right. For example, leukaemia in children was once always fatal. Many clinical trials have developed the excellent drug therapies that are now used with great success. However, a goal for public health and epidemiologists is to prevent children from ever developing this disease.

One of the early clues to the aetiology of the disease was from looking at the rates by age in the first few years of life. The incidence rises sharply from shortly after birth to a peak around the age of 4 years. Then there is a rapid decline in incidence to a very low level around the age of 14. These simple descriptive statistics may hold the clue to the cause. It has been hypothesized that early-life experiences, possibly infectious disease, may cause or facilitate the development of acute leukaemia in children.

Summary

Incidence rates are an important feature of epidemiology and measure the rate of occurrence of the outcome, the rate at which new cases are added to the prevalent pool. The population at risk must be defined and measured with respect to time. Person-years is the most common way to measure the volume of the population available to be an incident case.

Indirect and direct standardization is used to compare subgroups, or to compare between studies. Directly standardized rates use an external, standard, population to weight the average of the stratum-specific rates. Indirect rates are derived from the ratio of the observed and expected number of cases. The expected number of cases is derived from the overall rates of disease and the population in the specific stratum of the subgroup.

Self-test questions

Q 4.6.1: Which of these could be used as a stratum for calculating directly standardized incidence rates?
A Age
B Sex
C Ethnic group
D Geographical region
E Outcome
F Exposure

Q 4.6.2: The rates that use an external or standard population in their calculation are:
A Directly standardized rates
B Indirectly standardized rates
C Prevalence rates

Q 4.6.3: Sub-area rates within a study area may be compared using:
A Directly standardized rates
B Indirectly standardized rates

Q 4.6.4: In a study from a general practice there were 28 males and 47 females newly diagnosed with a form of eczema over the course of a year. There was a total of 2100 males and 2398 females registered at the mid-point in the year of study. What are the stratum-specific rates?

Q 4.6.5: From Question 4.6.4, what is the crude overall rate of this form of eczema?

4.7 Risk of Disease

- Pre-requisite sections: 2.1, 3.7, 3.8.
- Learning outcome: By the end of this section you should be able to define absolute and relative risk and interpret it.

In epidemiology we are interested in the likelihood of a particular outcome, for example the likelihood of a patient dying, of becoming obese, of having lung cancer, of being born premature. We can express likelihood in two ways: risk or odds. The risk of some event is synonymous with probability of an outcome, but epidemiology tends to use the word risk. The odds take a somewhat different form and are discussed in Section 4.8.

Risk may be expressed in absolute or relative terms. The relative form compares two or more groups and is known as a relative risk. In many epidemiology study designs, the interest focuses upon the risk of getting a disease amongst people exposed to a risk factor or treatment, compared to the risk of the disease when unexposed to the risk factor or treatment. It is not possible to measure risk in a case-control study, or a study of prevalence. Classically, cohort studies and RCTs measure the incidence of disease in a suitable population, which permits the calculation of risk.

Language in common use confuses the words probability and possibility. Possibility has two outcomes, either possible or not possible: where something is not possible it will not happen. Probability is a continuum between the two extremes of definitely will happen and definitely will not happen, and is a more realistic approach to representing the situation.

Risk will not inform an individual's cause

The risk for developing a disease, either in an absolute sense, or in relation to a risk factor should not be confused with attempting to assign a 'personal risk'. For example, it is not possible to decide whether a person's brain tumour was due to use of their mobile phone or due to some other cause. Box 4.7 explores this important point).

The personal risk of an outcome is 0% until the person develops the disease. At that point their probability is 100%: they definitely have the disease. For example what is a heavy smoker's risk of lung cancer? Heavy smokers have 10% lifetime risk of lung cancer. However, 90% of these have 0% risk and 10% of these have 100% risk. This gives an average risk of 10%.

Medical risk is more than science and statistics: it involves legal, spiritual and personal factors. The role played by risk is important in shared decision making, the approach where clinicians and patients communicate using the best available evidence when making decisions about their health, where the patient is supported to decide about the relative attributes and consequences of the various options available. The overarching aim is to arrive at an informed decision between the doctor and patient. Patients need information about risk, provided by their doctor. Patients also need to understand risk themselves and this requires meaningful two-way dialogue between the doctor and the patient.

Many laws place duties on clinicians regarding information disclosure such as risk, and there are also ethical standards. These require clarity over what is meant by the term 'risk'. A second part of shared decision making is that the understanding of risk to one person, such as the doctor, is a way of achieving a desirable goal, whilst to another, such as the patient, risk is something to avoid at all costs (see Box 4.8).

Absolute risk is the chance something happens

Absolute risk of disease, in simple terms, is the probability of disease. A probability ranges between one, which means an outcome is certain to happen, and zero, where we are certain an outcome will not happen. A patient with a disease has a risk of one for the disease already. The challenge presented to researchers and clinicians is to assess accurately the risks of a disease before the event. It is often easier to articulate, particularly to people not used to science, as a percentage ranging from 0% to 100%. A probability of 0.5, or 50%, means there is an equal chance of the event occurring as not. We measure absolute risk, AR, as the occurrence of new events, or cases, in a population:

$$AR = \frac{\text{Chance something happens}}{\text{Chance something happens} + \text{Chance nothing happens}}$$

To illustrate the estimation of risk let us consider a hospital-acquired infection. We begin by defining the infection carefully, and it might be defined as an infection that is documented by cultures, not incubated at admission, occurred at least 48 hours after admission and occurred no more than 48 hours following discharge. Using this series of definitions, we could examine cancer patients in a hospital as the population at risk. In our example we have records that show that 3019 cancer patients passed through the hospital in a certain period. These represent the total set of everything happening, which is the sum of the chance something and the chance nothing happens. Of these, 358 suffered a hospital-acquired infection: something happened. Therefore the risk of a hospital-acquired infection was:

$$AR = \frac{358}{3019} = 0.1186$$

This is interpreted as a risk of 11.86% for a cancer patient to acquire an infection during their stay in hospital.

Relative risk is used for causal modelling

Aetiological research needs to associate the risk of an outcome with factors or exposures that potentially may have caused that disease. One way of doing this is to estimate the relative risk of a disease due to an exposure. The relative risk is used in this case, instead of an absolute risk, because an event may take place in an unexposed or control group with no exposure to a putative risk factor under investigation. This may be due to chance alone, or other competing risks. For this reason the relative risk is a more useful measure than absolute risk for identifying risk facts and is defined as:

$$RR = \frac{\text{Risk in exposed group}}{\text{Risk in unexposed group}}$$

For many epidemiological studies, we measure the relative risk using a risk ratio. In cohort studies subgroups are selected by their exposure and observed over time, then risk of disease can be calculated. This allows a comparison of the risk of getting a disease between the exposed and unexposed groups. The randomized controlled trial compares the risk of the event, or outcome, between the controls, or unexposed group, and the treatment group. In its simplest terms, the proportion of the exposed that are cases, divided by the proportion of unexposed that are cases gives the risk ratio.

We begin by calculating the event rates, or rates of the outcome, in the exposed (EER) and unexposed (UER) groups as

$$EER = \frac{e_1}{e_0 + e_1}$$

and

$$UER = \frac{u_1}{u_0 + u_1}$$

where e_1 and e_0 are the number of cases and non-cases in the exposed group, and u_1 and u_0 are the number of cases and non-cases in the unexposed group respectively. The risk ratio (RR) is the ratio of these two event rates:

$$RR = \frac{EER}{UER}$$

A risk ratio is simple to interpret

A risk ratio of greater than one suggests the risk of the disease is associated with the risk factor. In other words, the proportion of people exposed to the putative risk factor who are cases is greater than in the non-case group. A risk ratio of less than one shows that the risk factor protects against the disease.

Let us illustrate this with the example given in Table 3.1. The risk of death, which is the event rate in the two groups, exposed to the intervention, aspirin, and unexposed, is

$$EER = \frac{38}{38 + 280} = 0.119$$

and

$$UER = \frac{42}{42 + 276} = 0.132$$

This shows that the risk of death, over the course of the trial, in the unexposed or control groups was approximately 13%, and in the intervention group was lower at 12%. The relative risk of death in the intervention group compared to the control group is

$$RR = \frac{0.119}{0.132} = 0.90$$

This suggests that there is a decreased risk of death in the aspirin, or intervention, group compared to the group not taking aspirin.

Clinicians and the public want to know risk reduction

The measure of relative risk is an important epidemiological measure. However, clinicians and policy makers wish to know whether the risk is reduced, and to what extent. One measure of this is the absolute risk reduction (ARR) and is calculated as

$$ARR = EER - UER$$

Sometimes we may wish to compare the risk reduction to the baseline risk, and this gives the relative risk reduction (RRR). This is given by

$$RRR = \frac{EER - UER}{UER}$$

Returning to our example of aspirin protecting against death (Table 3.1) this gives

$$ARR = 0.119 - 0.132 = -0.013$$

and

$$RRR = \frac{0.119 - 0.132}{0.132} = -0.095$$

which suggests that there will be a reduction in the rate of death of 0.013 persons per person taking aspirin. The RRR may be more useful in a clinical setting as it accounts for both the effectiveness of an intervention and for the relative likelihood of an event in the absence of the intervention. This shows that the risk of death, for a person taking aspirin, is reduced by 9.8% compared to not taking aspirin.

Absolute and relative risks provide different information

It is commonplace for the media to report the benefits of a new treatment for a disease, or how avoiding a certain aspect to our environment will prevent a disease. These are often presented as measures of relative risk reduction that do not account for the actual impact on health. However, a patient or member of the public will want to know how much it changes his or her own risk.

For example there may be a new drug which reduces the risk of developing a disease by 50%. This may seem important, but you must also take into account what the underlying absolute risk is. For example, were the risk equal to 2 in 10,000, then the drug would reduce the risk by only one person in every 10,000. This modest achievement must be weighed against the level of danger posed by the disease and any side-effects associated with the disease and policy makers must also look at cost.

Patient and doctor perspectives on risk

Meaningful discussion on risk helps ensure the validity of consent when patients decide to have an intervention, or not. Both the patient and doctor bring with them completely different attitudes and perceptions, reflecting a diverse range of views and perspectives about risk (see Box 4.8). On occasion, the views of patients might appear irrational to the doctor, but for patients with legal capacity, rationality is not the issue. An objective and indeed measurable judgement as to what is a rational view about risk is not possible at this time. To place this in perspective, crossing the road is sometimes more dangerous in terms of risk than having some medical tests. We often cross the road without any real thought or discussion with others, however medical interventions are often the subject for serious deliberation.

When clinicians avoid making unfounded assumptions about preferences and values held by their patients, misunderstandings about things important to patients and the harm they cause are avoided. Lawsuits are most often based on medical error and if a clinician can minimize errors in communication this can be an important first step (Studdert *et al.*, 2006). Patients may not understand the implications of what they are told, not remember what they were told, not be given the necessary information or not be given an opportunity to ask questions. The difficulties associated with decision making are highlighted in Box 4.9.

Decision making is difficult for patients. The characteristics of decision making in colorectal and lung cancer patients have been assessed (Keating *et al.*, 2010) and it was noted that if there was strong evidence then the doctor was more likely to share the decision making, that more patient control was seen in regards to chemotherapy treatment, and doctor control was more seen in regards to surgery and radiotherapy treatment. The expectations around patient preferences in metastatic disease usually involve less patient involvement.

Risk perception differs between specialties

Between disciplines, risk management may also differ. Anaesthetics look to assist rather than cure, so as a discipline, anaesthesiology is probably more risk averse than

---

Box 4.9. Centralization of services and risk

Internationally, cancer treatment services are concentrated in centres treating high volumes of patients and that offer a wide range of services, including surgery, oncology, radiotherapy, and specialized nursing and allied health services. These co-located comprehensive services with experienced staff can provide improved clinical outcomes for some patients when compared with centres that do not have the same level of experience or cannot provide the same services (Campbell *et al.*, 2006).

At present in colorectal cancer care most patients are managed by surgeons who treat a small number of patients. However there is considerable variation in the implementation of effective care within secondary care (Kelly *et al.*, 2003). At what point does the risk of receiving treatment in a low volume, non-specialist hospital become more important than receiving treatment quickly?

---

a specialty such as cardiothoracic surgery. Surgical interventions carry high levels of risk but which patients may nonetheless think is a risk worth taking because of the lack of alternatives.

Risk management, risk-based regulation and risk-benefit ratios all have meaning in the context of healthcare organization. But risk to a hospital manager is different to risk as a hospital patient understands it when making personal choices. The patient has to deal with technical information which can often be unfamiliar; while when published data is available, it can sometimes be inconclusive. Therefore the patients as well as the clinician both need a way of dealing with uncertainty.

Understanding risk relies on trust

Communication about risk tends to rely on reference to statistics, and this reliance may not help patients. While a doctor can inform a patient about a particular risk, the way in which information is presented can have a material bearing on the outcome of a decision. Doctors can sometimes tick a box indicating that a patient is sufficiently informed to make a choice. In reality, the patient may have an inadequate understanding of what they are signing up to because information was not framed in an appropriate way or did not take account of their personal values.

Why is this important? Often the patient has a high level of concern regarding their health. Other barriers include a low level of trust in the individual who may be thought of by the patient as representing a larger organization that does not have the best interests of the patient at heart. Within the healthcare environment there are differential relationships of power, where the patient often feels powerless.

Trust is important here. Establishing trust can be in the form of third party endorsements from credible sources, demonstrating to the patient the supporting characteristics, by showing caring, honesty and consistency. The nature of the information communicated is often complex with uncertainty or expert disagreement. It is this point that may undermine a patient's trust in an intervention or a healthcare professional. Science is about disproving something; a science success is disproving something that until then had been considered by the public as true. This change in the knowledge base is difficult for a patient to understand.

Communicating risk is difficult

Effective risk communication involves the clinician knowing why they are communicating the information. Distinctions between outcomes are important; however, the processes involved in reaching these outcomes can be equally important for patients. By identifying and understanding a patient's concerns, beliefs and perceptions, communication can be improved, as good risk communication is two-way. Effective communication requires knowing the patient as a person, which enables the clinician to understand the patient's problems and concerns from their perspective.

Risk perceptions are related to health behaviour, medical-decision making and the processing of health information. Patients' risk perception is influenced by a wide variety of cognitive, motivational and affective factors and these psychological processes often lead to errors in risk perception among laypeople, and the media in particular. Simply providing your truth or supplemental information does not cure what a clinician perceives as 'wrong' perceptions.

It is not desirable or practical to inform all patients of all and every conceivable eventuality of interacting with a healthcare organization. Judgement must be employed when deciding how much information about risk to communicate. Judgement is also required when deciding which patient is informed and the process by which they are informed. However, the litigation society has led drug companies to list every possible side-effect reported for a drug. These are often long lists of symptoms and are sometimes unproven as caused by the drug. The result is often the patient experiencing some fear regarding the drug.

Risk is multi-dimensional

Simple representations between an expert and patient may not be the best way to capture what is happening. Risk equations entail questions about severity and probability, as well as timing. The content and process differ significantly. When assessing risk, an expert uses scientific method, probabilistic measures and a concept of acceptable risk that goes beyond a single patient. In addition, the expert has a changing knowledge, whereby comparative risk can be known, as are population averages and a detachment from adverse events.

The patient on the other hand uses a more intuitive and often categorical way of making sense of the world. An answer to a question is either yes or no, and it either is or is not. Patients often see events as discrete while the weight of personal consequences is heavy. The detachment is lost and the process can be as important as the outcome especially in terms of palliative care. It matters how we die.

Risk of harm

A broader question of what constitutes harm needs consideration. The range of possible complications extends from death at one extreme to mild and temporary discomfort at the other, with short-term consequences in between with varying degrees of pain and disability. Poor clinical outcomes are bad for patients as well as for providers; poor outcomes that are unanticipated can be more significant than anticipated outcomes, especially when it comes to questions of liability. Clinical judgement needs to accommodate patient-centred values and preferences when dealing with questions of risk, and the ethics of risk are just as important as the science and the law when it comes to decisions about how much information of what kind is disclosed to which patients and when.

Summary

Risk is an important concept for epidemiologists, public health, clinicians and patients. It may be expressed in relative or absolute terms, each having a place but both having problems for interpretation. Absolute risk is the chance that something happens. Relative risk is a comparison of absolute risks between two groups, for example patients exposed to a putative risk factor and those not exposed.

The cause of disease in an individual will not be known with certainty; this is based on a range from 0 to 100%. Patients and the public want to know how this relates to them. Communication of risk is very difficult and involves other issues in addition to statistics.

Self-test questions

Q 4.7.1: What pieces of information do we need to calculate the relative risk reduction?

Q 4.7.2: A risk estimate that compares two groups is known as:
A Absolute risk
B Relative risk
C Relative risk reduction

Q 4.7.3: A cohort study compared people living in cold houses to people living in warm houses in relation to hypertension. The investigators found that 468 people were in warm houses and 445 in cold houses. In the cold houses there were 232 people diagnosed with hypertension, and there were a total of 386 people overall diagnosed with hypertension. What is the relative risk?

Q 4.7.4: How do you interpret the estimate of relative risk in Q 4.7.3?

4.8   Odds and Odds Ratios

- Pre-requisite sections: 2.1, 3.6, 4.7.
- Learning outcome: By the end of this section you should be able to calculate and interpret an odds ratio.

In a cohort study or a randomized controlled trial we measure the number of people with an outcome, in relation to the population from which they were sampled. However, for a case-control study, we do not sample cases and non-cases, known as controls, in proportion to their distribution in the underlying population. This is a strength of the design: for rare diseases we directly recruit cases of the disease rather than waiting for them to appear in the cohort or trial.

Odds is calculated for a case-control study

This leads to a difficulty: we are no longer able to calculate risk, as the ratio of the numerator, the cases, and the denominator, the population, is biased through the selection and recruitment method. The epidemiologist must find a different method of calculating relative risk from a case-control study; instead of risk, the case-control study uses odds.

The probability, or risk, of a particular outcome happening can be defined as the number of outcomes divided by the total number of possible outcomes. The odds of an event are slightly different; they are the number of times the event occurs, the chance something happens, divided by the number of times it does not occur. In terms of probability and chance:

$$Odds = \frac{\text{Chance something happens}}{\text{Chance something does not happen}}$$

The odds of disease in the exposed group are:

$$Odds = \frac{e_1}{e_0}$$

where e_1 and e_0 are the number of exposed cases and controls respectively. The odds for disease in the unexposed group are:

$$Odds = \frac{u_1}{u_0}$$

where u_1 and u_0 are the number of unexposed cases and controls respectively.

Odds ratio estimates the relative risk

The risk-based study designs, such as the cohort study, measure association between the outcome and the exposure using the risk ratio. The case-control study can estimate odds, not risk, and so has a different measure known as the odds ratio, often abbreviated to OR. The odds ratio is given by the ratio of these two odds:

$$OR = \frac{e_1}{e_0} \bigg/ \frac{u_1}{u_0}$$

Using an example to illustrate these measures, let us imagine we wish to estimate who is more likely to drink beer before noon: students or teachers? Is one group more likely to drink beer before noon on a given day? Table 4.4 shows some data collected on whether a person drinks before noon or doesn't drink before noon which is the outcome we are interested in. The explanatory variable is whether the person is a student or a teacher.

The odds of a student drinking before noon is:

$$Odds = \frac{45}{5} = 9 : 1$$

The odds of a teacher drinking beer before noon is:

$$Odds = \frac{10}{40} = 0.25 : 1$$

Table 4.4. Number of people in a case-control study of drinking beer between teachers and students.

	Drink beer	Do not drink beer	Total
Student	45	5	50
Teacher	10	40	50
Total	55	45	100

Therefore the odds ratio is

$$OR = \frac{45}{5} \Big/ \frac{10}{40} = 36$$

How do we interpret the odds ratio?

If the odds ratio equals one, there is no effect, no association between the outcome and the exposure or risk factor. In other words, the exposure does not cause the disease. If the odds ratio is greater than one, then we say that there is an association. The exposure raises the risk of disease. Alternatively, the odds ratio may be less than one, and the converse applies. There is still an association, but the exposure lowers the risk of disease or protects against that disease.

Returning to the example above, the odds ratio was very large at 36. This may be interpreted as students have a higher odds of drinking before noon than their teachers. We may also equate this with the risk, and infer that the risk is also increased.

A more detailed example

Imagine we wish to explore the types and extent of eating difficulties and the need for assistance when eating, in patients admitted for stroke rehabilitation over a period of one year. The outcome variable is dependent feeding for people who eat less than three quarters of served food (Westergren *et al.*, 2001). The data are shown in Table 4.5.

We can calculate the odds of dependent feeding in people who do not eat three quarters or less of served food as

$$Odds = \frac{17}{44} = 0.386$$

The odds ratio for dependent feeding in people who do and those who do not eat three quarters or less of served food is

$$OR = \frac{59}{33} \Big/ \frac{17}{44} = 4.63$$

This odds ratio is greater than one and we conclude that people who eat three quarters or less of served food are at increased risk of dependent feeding. This is important as by systematically assessing for eating difficulties we may help to facilitate eating,

Table 4.5. Study of the types and extent of eating difficulties and the need for assistance when eating in patients admitted for stroke rehabilitation.

	Dependent	Independent	Total
Eating three quarters or less	59	33	92
Eating more than three quarters	17	44	61
Total	76	77	153

especially as patients with eating difficulties risk becoming undernourished and developing pressure ulcers.

Odds ratio is similar to risk ratio for rare diseases

As we can see, the odds ratio is not exactly the same number as the risk ratio. This is because we do not know the risk. A simple rule-of-thumb is that the odds ratio becomes closer to the risk ratio as the disease becomes rare. There is, however, no magic number at which point the odds ratio becomes acceptable.

We can see how this works, through a straightforward examination of the symbols. Remember, the risk ratio is the ratio of the event rates, or rates of the outcome, in the exposed (EER) and unexposed (UER) groups:

$$EER = \frac{e_1}{e_0 + e_1}$$

and

$$UER = \frac{u_1}{u_0 + u_1}$$

where e_1 and e_0 are the number of cases and non-cases in the exposed group, and u_1 and u_0 are the number of cases and non-cases in the unexposed group respectively. The risk ratio is:

$$RR = \frac{EER}{UER} = \frac{e_1}{e_0 + e_1} \bigg/ \frac{u_1}{u_0 + u_1}$$

The ratio of the odds used for calculating the odds ratio is:

$$OR = \frac{e_1}{e_0} \bigg/ \frac{u_1}{u_0}$$

As you can see by these two equations, as the number of cases, the e_1 and u_1, becomes a smaller and smaller number, the value of the event rates (EER and UER) approach the same value as the odds. Therefore the odds ratio approaches the risk ratio.

If this does not convince you, then Fig. 4.10 shows a series of case-control studies where the underlying risk ratio is three. The calculated odds ratio is not exactly the same as the risk ratio; as the proportion of the population who are cases increases so the odds ratio becomes further and further from the risk ratio. Also note that the odds ratio does not replicate the risk ratio in this example. The differences between odds and risk are highlighted in Box 4.10 using the odds seen at the races.

Summary

The odds ratio is designed for use in studies where the risk cannot be calculated, such as the case-control study. Instead the odds of the outcome can be calculated and this is an approximation of the risk ratio. For this reason it is seen as a measure of relative risk. As the outcome, or disease, becomes rarer, so the odds ratio approaches the risk ratio.

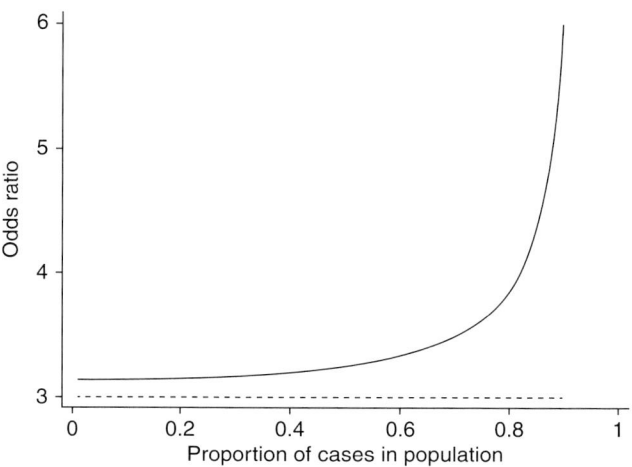

Fig. 4.10. A comparison of how the odds ratio deviates from the risk ratio as the disease becomes more common.

Box 4.10. Odds and probability

The term 'odds' is used by bookmakers for horse racing, and when a bookmaker offers odds of '50 to one' that a horse will win the next race, the odds are one divided by 50, or 0.02. If you placed £1 on a horse, a real outsider, at an odds of 50 to one, you would get back £51 (at the races you get your initial bet back as well if you win).

The probability of your horse winning is calculated as one divided by 51, which is practically the same as the odds. This is also relevant for epidemiology: for a rare disease, which is equivalent to the long odds on our horse above, the odds and the probability of disease are very close. But when the disease is common, let's say odds of four to one, this gives odds of 25% but a probability, or risk, of 20%, which are different.

However, the epidemiologist should be aware of the problems with the odds ratio when used for measuring relative risk.

Self-test questions

Q 4.8.1: The odds ratio for Benny's Bistro was 2.46. Which of the following would be a correct interpretation of this odds ratio?

A 2.46% of the people who ate food from Benny's Bistro developed food poisoning

B The incidence of food poisoning among people who ate food from the bistro was 2.46/1000

C The odds that a 'case' ate at the Bistro were 2.46 to 1

D People who ate food from the Bistro had 2.46 times the risk of developing food poisoning compared to people who did not eat food from the Bistro

Q 4.8.2: The odds ratio is not appropriate for:
A Common diseases
B Rare diseases

Q 4.8.3: A case-control study identified 200 cases, with 145 participating. Of these 68 were exposed, whilst in the controls 24 were exposed. What information is missing?

Q 4.8.4: For Q 4.8.3, there was exactly one control for each case. What is the odds ratio?

Q 4.8.5: How do you interpret the odds ratio you obtained in Q 4.8.4?

4.9 Hypothesis Testing

- Pre-requisite sections: 1.2, 1.4, 4.3–4.8.
- Learning outcome: By the end of the section you should be able to describe using statistics in hypothesis testing.

Scientific method proceeds with the declaration of a hypothesis that the scientist aims to reject. But how does the scientist reject a hypothesis? One way is by the epidemiologist designing a study that addresses the question, data is collected and this is then statistically analysed to test the hypothesis.

Statistical distributions are smooth curves

We will begin with statistical distributions. A histogram presents a frequency distribution of observations in a study. Now imagine that a very large number of observations were made, and that the widths of the histogram classes are made very small. When the number of observations approaches infinity and the histogram bin widths shrink to zero, the outline of the histogram would then look like the underlying, 'theoretical' distribution. It would probably be a smooth line, rather than composed of steps in the data. This is demonstrated in Fig. 4.11.

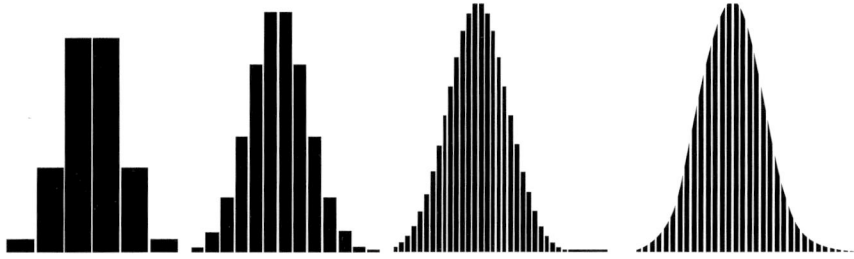

Fig. 4.11. Histogram of frequency distribution with bin widths shrinking.

The theoretical distribution can take many different forms, but the most important, and most common for numeric continuous data, is known as the 'normal distribution', also known as the 'Gaussian distribution' or the 'bell curve' as it resembles a bell shape. The greatest frequency of observations occurs at the same point, the centre of the distribution which is also the mean, median and mode value. The standard deviation of the distribution describes how broad the bell shape is, and the horizontal axis represents the values taken by the variable.

Statistical distributions can be used to estimate the probability of a measure

If a variable can be regarded as having a normal distribution, and the mean and variance are known, then the probability of any value of the variable can be calculated. Figure 4.12 shows a distribution of 1000 observations with a mean of 163 and a standard deviation of 6. A normally distributed line has been superimposed on the figure. A plot like this may, for example, represent the height of patients in a clinic on the x-axis, where the mean height is 163 cm and the standard deviation is 6 cm. In the plot, the y-axis, or vertical axis, is the count or frequency of patients for each height.

Figure 4.12 is approximately normally distributed and the knowledge of this distribution allows us to make statements about the probability of finding different values of the variable. To help us do this the total area under the normal curve is usually defined as 1.0: one whole unit. We know that the proportion of people taller than 163 cm (and indeed less than 163 cm) is 0.5 (50%), as this is the centre of the normal distribution. The probability that a normal random variable is greater than its mean is 0.5, and the probability that it is less than its mean is 0.5.

We may also use known characteristics of the normal distribution to state how many patients have a height greater than 165 cm. Technically the chance of finding a patient who is precisely 165 cm, that is not 165.000000001 cm and not 164.999999999 cm is very remote, and so of no interest. In this case the probability

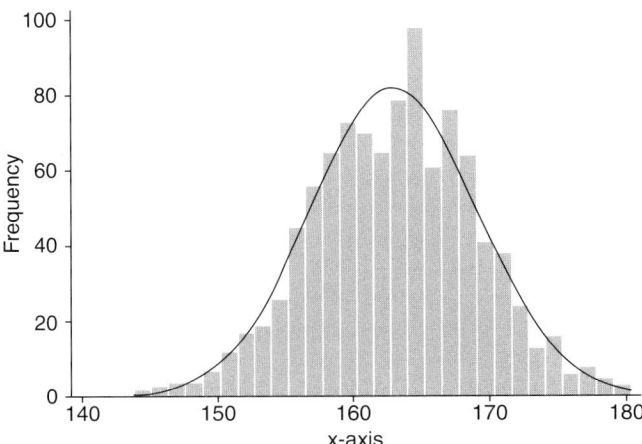

Fig. 4.12. Histogram of heights, with a mean of 163 and standard deviation of 6.

that a patient, if selected at random, is taller than 165 cm is 0.37. This is the proportion of the area under the normal curve, compared to the whole curve, to the right of 165 in the figure. That is 37% of the total area is right of the value of 165.

Only the standard normal is required

It is neither possible, nor necessary, to tabulate the areas under normal curves for all possible combinations of mean and standard deviation. All normal curves have the same bell shape and just one 'standard normal' curve is tabulated. All we need to know is the mean and standard deviation of the data. The standard curve has a mean of zero and standard deviation of one.

To make probability statements about any normal variable, it is necessary to 'transform' it to a standard normal. To do this, for any value in the distribution you subtract the mean, and then divide by the standard deviation. The mathematical equation, which we will refer to as z, is:

$$z = \frac{x - \bar{x}}{SD}$$

where x is the value transformed to a standard normal variable, with $\bar{x}$ and SD the mean and standard deviation of the distribution respectively. For the example above, the mean height is 163 cm and standard deviation 6 cm. So a height of 165 cm is transformed as follows:

1. Subtract the mean of 163 from the value

   $165 - 163 = 2$

2. Divide by the standard deviation of 6 to get

   $z = 2 / 6 = 0.33$

The value calculated above allows the area to the left of the point to be determined by looking the value up in a table, or more probably using statistical software. The area under the curve for a value where z is less than, or equal to, 0.33 is 0.6293. Since the total area under the curve is one, the probability that a value is greater than $z = 0.33$ is $1 - 0.6293 = 0.3707$. Consequently the probability that a patient selected at random is taller than 165 cm is 0.37 (or 37%).

Hypothesis testing begins with defining the hypothesis

The first formal step in hypothesis testing is to state the hypothesis. We most commonly begin with the 'null' hypothesis and the 'alternative' hypothesis. The null hypothesis, traditionally referred to as 'H0', is chosen to assume no effect. Thus if a drug is tested, the null hypothesis will be that the drug has no effect. In medical statistics it is better, and almost always the case, to assume the alternative hypothesis (known as H1 or Ha) to be 'two-sided'. This means, that if there is an effect, that effect may be beneficial or harmful. There would be two one-sided hypotheses, one would be that the effect were beneficial, and the other harmful.

As an example, consider a study in which 400 women with hypertension are prescribed a new anti-hypertensive treatment. Systolic blood pressure is measured before the treatment and then again after the course of treatment and changes in blood pressure are recorded. The null hypothesis will be that the mean change in blood pressure is zero: the treatment has no effect. The alternative hypothesis will be that the mean change is not zero: the mean change is either less than zero (the pressure has reduced and the drug is considered beneficial) or greater than zero (the drug is considered harmful). This is a two-sided hypothesis.

Scientists define errors for the hypothesis testing

When a scientist decides to test a hypothesis they must define two parameters. The first, alpha (α) traditionally set at 0.05, is the probability of a type I error. A type I error is the probability of rejecting the null hypothesis when the null hypothesis is actually true, also known as a false negative. The probability of accepting the null hypothesis when it is true is equal to $1 - \alpha$.

The second parameter to be defined is beta (β), the probability of a type II error, which is the probability of not rejecting a false null hypothesis or a false positive. This is known as the 'power' of a study which is its ability to detect what we are looking for. These different errors will be used in many situations, such as calculating a required sample size, and conducting statistical testing.

Statistical testing generates a p-value

The statistician will then define a statistical test of the null hypothesis; the choice of test statistic will depend on the situation. Using the blood pressure example, there will be 400 differences in blood pressure. The null hypothesis was that there would be no change and therefore a mean change of 0 mmHg. In this example there was a mean change of 1 mmHg, which is small but possibly the drug is having an impact. However, the standard deviation from the sample was 11 mmHg.

The concept of standard deviation was introduced to describe spread, which was important for the normal distribution. The spread of the mean of the measurements, not the spread of the actual measurements, is given by the 'standard error' or the 'standard error of the mean'. There is a relationship between the standard deviation (SD) of the population and the standard error of the sample mean (SE) taking into account the sample size (n). This is given by:

$$SE = \frac{SD}{\sqrt{n}}$$

In our example the standard deviation of the systolic blood pressure is 11 mmHg, the standard error of the mean of a sample of size 40 is 1.74 mmHg. When the sample size increases to 400, the standard error reduces to 0.55 mmHg.

This test allows us to generate a z-value which was introduced earlier. This time, as we are interested in the difference of a mean from a value, we must use the standard error of the mean (SE) rather than the standard deviation.

$$z = \frac{x - \bar{x}}{SE}$$

The z-value can be obtained and related to the normal distribution to obtain a p-value. This is the probability that, assuming the null hypothesis is true, you would obtain this test statistic. This requires a cut-off, defined by the α, which is traditionally set to 0.05 or less. When the p-value is less than α the analyst can state that the null hypothesis is rejected, and the alternative hypothesis is statistically significant. This is not the same as saying that the p-value is the probability that the null hypothesis is true.

Interpreting the p-value

It is common to misinterpret the p-value, some examples of how are outlined in Box 4.11. Returning to our example, the z-value is

$$z = \frac{1 - 0}{0.55} = 1.82$$

Relating this to the z table, this gives a p-value of 0.07, which is greater than our defined cut-off of 0.05. The interpretation is that, assuming that the null hypothesis is true, the probability of getting a z-value at least as extreme as the one obtained is 0.07. In advance, we chose an alpha of 0.05, and this suggests that you cannot reject the null hypothesis, and therefore infer that the drug has no effect on the blood pressure.

There are many other hypothesis tests

We have so far introduced a simple test of significance, the z-test. There are many other tests, each addressing different situations. The situations may be different types of data, such as qualitative or quantitative, or shapes of distributions such as normal or bi-modal. The analyst must use their skills and experience to determine the type of test required for the situation.

A common, simple and yet powerful test, the 'Student's t-test', was developed to deal with normally distributed data such as gathered from the blood pressure study. The test defines a value of t. A p-value may then be generated. A different test is more appropriate for categorical data, or data that is not normally distributed. One of these tests is known as the χ^2 test (in English spelt 'chi-squared', and pronounced 'ki-squared', with a hard 'k' and rhymes with 'why'). This allows a comparison of the count of the observed data and that which would be expected. This will also generate a p-value.

Summary

An epidemiology study is designed to follow the scientific method, which involves testing a hypothesis. To test a hypothesis, the analyst begins by defining a null

Box 4.11. Hypothetically speaking

The researchers in a new paper have deduced that there is a difference between the treatment and the control group in their study. They reached this conclusion because the p-value was 0.001, which is less than 0.05. But how do we interpret this? Some common misinterpretations are that:

- It shows that the probability that the null hypothesis is true is one in 1000.
- It shows that the probability that the alternative hypothesis is true is 0.999.
- The p-value is very small and so the effect must be strong.

The first isn't quite correct, and the second is the first the other way around (also not correct). In terms of the strength of the effect, there is a relationship between the two, but you cannot deduce the strength of the effect from the p-value.

The correct way to interpret the p-value is that it is the probability of obtaining the test statistic at least as extreme as the one that was obtained, assuming that the null hypothesis is true.

hypothesis, and tries to reject this using some form of statistical test. The z-test uses the normal distribution to generate a p-value. There are other statistical tests that use different distributions. The p-value must be interpreted with care, and should not be used as a report of the effect of the factor being tested.

Self-test questions

Q 4.9.1: True or false? The standard deviation is always smaller than, or equal to, the standard error.

Q 4.9.2: The z-test needs which of the following?
A Mean
B Standard deviation
C Number of observations
D Odds ratio
E Type I error level (alpha)
F Type II error level (beta)
G p-value

Q 4.9.3: The z-score of the mean blood pressure for 400 participants in a study is:
A Greater than a z-score for 4000 participants
B Less than a z-score for 4000 participants
C The same as a z-score for 4000 participants

4.10 Confidence Intervals

- Pre-requisite sections: 1.2, 1.4, 4.3–4.9.
- Learning outcome: By the end of the section you should be able to describe confidence intervals and give their interpretation.

Many journals and epidemiologists prefer not to see articles relying on p-values to make inference. They prefer to see a 'confidence interval' quoted: a range of values, an interval, within which the true value is likely to lie. The importance of confidence intervals for clinicians is highlighted in Box 4.12, exploring differently sized trials of a drug.

Confidence intervals are used to test hypotheses, in a similar way to the p-value. When a scientist wishes to test a null hypothesis, such as whether a change in blood pressure is zero, then the confidence interval could be used to ask whether it contains the null hypothesis. The confidence interval for the true population mean, $\bar{x}$, is given by the lower (LCI) and upper (UCI) bounds, defined as:

$$UCI = \bar{x} + (\Phi SE)$$

and

$$LCI = \bar{x} - (\Phi SE)$$

where the standard error of the mean (SE) and a critical value theta (Φ) are used to find the bounds.

Confidence intervals are based on a percentage

The most commonly quoted confidence interval is the 95% confidence interval, which represents the interval within which the measure of location in 95% of similar studies would lie. This can be changed to a 99% confidence interval, which is wider than the 95% interval, or narrowed for say an 80% confidence interval. This means that when you are judging whether a value lies outside of the confidence interval, a 99% confidence interval is more stringent than the 95% confidence interval as it is a wider interval, and the opposite for an 80% confidence interval.

In order to specify confidence intervals it is necessary to look up critical values from a distribution, and the normal distribution is the most commonly used. When

---

Box 4.12. Experiment with confidence

Thinking back to the court case example in Box 4.4, it highlights a serious message: how do you know what you prescribe is the correct thing to give to your patient? We have been discussing how to deal with uncertainty and risk, which is certainly important. Here is a thought experiment to take into account sample sizes as well:

Imagine there is a randomized controlled trial. It seems to be well conducted. The active arm has three successes out of four in total and the control arm has two out of four. The risk reduction is 50%. Now – do you prescribe?

It is unlikely, as there are too few patients in this trial: just eight people in total. What about a study with 20 in each arm with the same risk reduction? Is it still too small? What about a study with 50, or 100, or 500, or 1000? At what point would you prescribe?

There is no point at which a study is sufficiently large to direct a clinician to prescribe. This is where the confidence interval steps in: it helps the clinician know whether to prescribe or not.

the standard deviation is somehow known for the data, or is estimated on a sample with 200 or more observations, we use a value, Φ, from the standard normal distribution. For example, in order to calculate the 95% confidence interval, we see that 2.5% of the standard normal distribution is smaller than $\Phi = -1.96$ and 2.5% of the distribution is greater than $\Phi = +1.96$. This means that 95% of the distribution lies between these two values. Commonly used confidence intervals give the following values of Φ: 80% –1.28 to +1.28; 90% –1.64 to +1.64; 95% –1.96 to +1.96; 99% –2.58 to +2.58.

Interpreting the confidence interval

This confidence interval can be interpreted as follows: if this study is repeated many times, a percentage of the times this interval will include the true value. When the 95% confidence interval is used then this percentage will be 95. The important role of the confidence interval is that it gives a feasible range of values within which the true population might lie. However, the confidence interval does not predict that the true value has a 95% probability of lying within the interval.

Consider an example where a treatment for hypertension causes a mean drop of systolic blood pressure of 20 mmHg. The point estimate at face value looks good. If however the 95% confidence interval for the mean is –10 to 50 mmHg then it should be noted that the drop may feasibly take the value of zero and therefore be of no value, or even be a rise in systolic blood pressure, that is the treatment could be harmful rather than beneficial. It is also true that the treatment might feasibly be better than the mean of 20 mmHg indicates. The simple truth is that the trial has not precisely determined the mean drop in systolic blood pressure and therefore further evidence should be sought before drawing conclusions about this treatment.

Small number of observations uses the Student's t-distribution

Where the standard deviation has been estimated from a sample with fewer than 200 observations, the critical values used to construct the confidence intervals will be a little bit larger. Rather than using the standard normal distribution, the Student's t-distribution should be used. Student's t is a little 'fatter' than the normal distribution. Figure 4.13 shows how the t-value approaches the z-value, for the 2.5% cut-off we use for 95% confidence intervals, as the number of observations increases.

A confidence interval for a prevalence

As the prevalence (P) is a proportion, and to calculate the standard error (SE) for use in the calculation of the confidence interval we use the standard error of a proportion:

$$SE = \sqrt{\frac{P(1-P)}{n}}$$

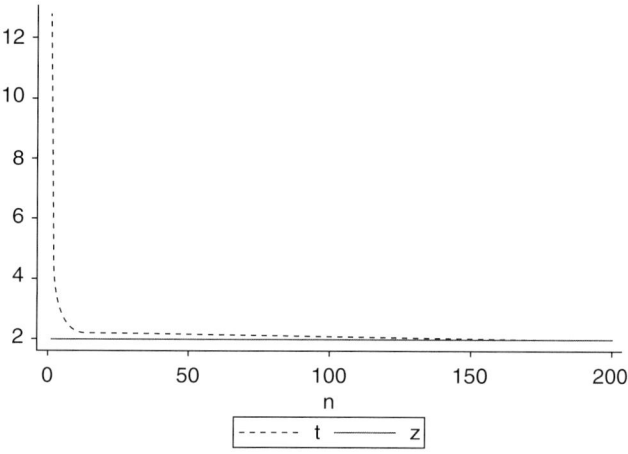

Fig. 4.13. Plot of t-values and z-values, for a p-value of 0.05, as the number of observations (n) increases.

where n is the number of people included in the sample. The upper (UCI) and lower (LCI) bounds of the confidence interval are, respectively:

$$UCI = P + (\alpha \times SE) \;\; and \;\; LCI = P - (\alpha \times SE)$$

where α was set by the epidemiologist.

A confidence interval for a risk ratio is symmetric on the log scale

Let us remind ourselves of the risk ratio (RR):

$$RR = \frac{e_1}{e_0 + e_1} \Big/ \frac{u_1}{u_0 + u_1}$$

where e_1 and e_0 are the number of cases and non-cases in the exposed group, and u_1 and u_0 are the number of cases and non-cases in the unexposed group respectively.

The risk ratio is normally distributed on the log scale, and so it is possible to calculate the confidence interval using the log of the risk ratio as the point estimate. The confidence interval is symmetric around the log of the risk ratio, with the upper (UCI) and lower (LCI) bounds calculated as:

$$\log(UCI) = \log(RR) + (\Phi \times SE(\log(RR))) \;\; and \;\; \log(LCI) = \log(RR) - (\Phi \times SE(\log(RR)))$$

The standard error for the log of the risk ratio is approximately:

$$SE\,(\log(RR)) = \sqrt{\frac{1}{e_1} + \frac{1}{u_1} - \frac{1}{e_0 + e_1} - \frac{1}{u_0 + u_1}}$$

The exponential can be taken of the lower and upper bounds of the confidence interval around the risk ratio.

The confidence interval for the odds ratio is similar to the rate ratio

In the same way as for the risk ratio, which is used for cohort studies and randomized controlled trials, the log of the odds ratio is normally distributed. The upper (UCI) and lower (LCI) confidence intervals are:

$$\log(UCI) = \log(OR) + (\Phi \times SE(\log(OR)))$$

and

$$\log(LCI) = \log(OR) - (\Phi \times SE(\log(OR)))$$

The standard error for the log of the odds ratio is approximately:

$$SE\ (\log\ OR) = \sqrt{\frac{1}{e_1} + \frac{1}{u_1} + \frac{1}{e_0} + \frac{1}{u_0}}$$

The confidence interval for the odds ratio is interpreted in the same way as for that calculated for the risk ratio. In simple terms, when the 95% confidence interval does not contain one, the odds ratio can be said to be statistically significantly different from the null hypothesis.

Summary

The confidence interval is used by scientists to determine whether a result, such as a mean, odds ratio, risk ratio or incidence rate is different from a null hypothesis. The confidence interval varies by the percentage that is required, the number of observations and the point estimate around which it is being calculated.

Self-test questions

Q 4.10.1: A case-control study found an odds ratio of 3.8, with a 95% confidence interval of 0.96 to 7.3. What can be deduced?

Q 4.10.2: True or false? The 95% confidence interval is wider than the 99% confidence interval.

Q 4.10.3: In a study of the prevalence of asthma in a GP surgery, the researcher discovered that in their practice population of 4876, there were 190 people with a record of symptoms of asthma. What is the prevalence and 95% confidence interval?

Q 4.10.4: The rate ratios from a cohort study are normally distributed on which scale?
A Linear scale
B Log scale

Further Reading

Bernhardt, V.L. (1998) *Multiple Measures*, Invited Monograph No. 4. California Association for Supervision and Curriculum Development (CASCD).

5 What Can Go Wrong: Error, Bias and Confounding

It has been said that the majority of an epidemiologist's job is to reduce bias. Sometimes this is how it feels. This chapter is designed to introduce the issues of error and bias.

5.1 Types of Error and Bias

- Pre-requisite sections: 1.2, 1.4, 1.5.
- Learning outcome: By the end of this section you should be able to describe error and bias and how an epidemiologist deals with them.

Some standard definitions for error and bias are as follows. Error is the difference between an estimated or measured value and the true value. Bias is 'systematic, non-random deviation of results and inferences from the truth, or processes leading to such a deviation' (Last, 2000).

These definitions hide a number of distractions though, which gives rise to them having different meanings to different people. Often these words have negative connotations, and sometimes for this reason researchers avoid discussing them. They do not want to be associated with a perceived weakness. However, it is important that as an epidemiologist you use tools that help you examine your work, and that of others, for potential sources of error and bias. This allows science to progress. Ignorance of these issues has led, and will in the future lead, to incorrect conclusions being drawn from health research.

Dealing with error and bias in science is usually free from the need to allocate blame, such as that more commonly associated with error in medical practice. Freedom from the 'blame game' makes the identification of bias, error and confounding an exercise in advancement, satisfying scientific curiosity and improving healthcare interventions and broader policy.

Observation provides the starting point

In the past the development of theories based on intuition and philosophy was the dominant approach to determining practice and policy: observation took a back seat. Hippocrates (circa 460–370 BC) set the basis for the empirical sciences, highlighting the need for observation and trial. We make observations and ensure these are as close to the truth as possible in order to make correct inferences. Francis Bacon (1561–1626) provided the method for the modern science experiment. He stated that a planned procedure was required. This starting point had freedoms such as attaching no blame, and it built on the insights and understanding that other philosophers had made with the aim to highlight the cause of things in the world.

Given philosophy has provided so much, what else can we learn about bias and error from philosophers? From the work of Immanuel Kant (1724–1804), professor of philosophy in Prussia, we can take the benefits of combining rational thought with experience: the thinking and the doing parts of experience. This avoids any error that could come from experience if it was just a hallucination. If we were just a 'brain in a vat' (see Box 5.1) then there would be no way of working out if what we were experiencing was real or just the application of a probe to an area of our brain to stimulate a particular experience.

One way of thinking about this is to imagine a scenario where we question the truths we hold when we are measuring something. Do they still hold true when we are not around to measure them? So again the epidemiologist's job is to work with the hypotheses generated and test them. These can be based on observation, intuition or experience in the field. Testing a hypothesis requires us to design, conduct and analyse the results of a study. The assumptions we make and the things we do in testing them are all places where bias and error can be introduced into the process of scientific enquiry.

Error is inherent in science and nature

One of the definitions of error is the difference between a measured value and what the value truly is. For this reason, error is inherent in biological systems and therefore in science. Indeed this error is exploited by nature, for example evolution requires errors to be made in reproduction to create the diversity needed to allow a species to change. This is analogous to a scientist's view of error, where their intention of perfect measurement is not met but they can benefit from the experience.

It is interesting to contrast error with fault. Fault implies culpability, which we are not interested in. An epidemiologist is interested in identifying and controlling for error, however it got there in the first place.

There is no simple way to spot error

Whether the study was conducted by someone else, or by you, the best approach to spotting error and bias is to be sceptical about everything. A quote from Peter Medawar helps us understand the importance of this sort of attitude: 'Before he sets out to convince others of his observations or opinions, a scientist must first convince himself. Let this not be too easily achieved; it is better by far to have the reputation

---

Box 5.1. 'Brain in a vat'

The brain in a vat is a thought experiment used by philosophy to examine the ideas of experience and reality. It proposes that a scientist puts a brain in a container (the vat) and connects it to electrodes. The brain would not know whether it was in a vat or in a skull.

---

for being querulous and unwilling to be convinced than to give reason to be thought gullible.' (Peter Brian Medawar, 1979).

How do we know that the study estimates of risk are accurate? Referring to the counterfactual approach to causation, we need to know if the study estimates are the same as the true values. Without a counterfactual situation we can't know this, the true study estimates are unknowable. We are left to try to reduce the bias we either guess or know exists.

Therefore the epidemiologist is left with needing to know where bias may exist. Using Fig. 5.1 you can go through the aspects of the study that may contain bias. However, even once you have gone through these possibilities, there is no substitute for thinking.

Removing error in a study

One of the most important decisions that is required by an epidemiologist is the design of the study. There are many advantages and disadvantages inherent in each design and these must be taken into account when determining how to investigate a scientific research question.

Following this, researchers must determine how they wish to collect the data and any other materials, such as biological samples, required during the data collection phase. There is considerable expertise and experience in designing data collection tools, such as questionnaires. Error may creep in at many points during this process and expert advice should be sought.

Other areas of the research process that are often ignored include the management of data and how the data is measured on individuals. Careful attention should be paid to the potential for human error being incorporated into any study data. At the data analysis phase there are potential sources of error even at this point. Using statistical techniques the epidemiologist now has the opportunity to reduce or ameliorate the effects of error in the study.

Steps to improve accuracy and precision

The first step that must be taken for reducing error is to clearly and concisely define the objectives of the research. This will include many decisions about what you want

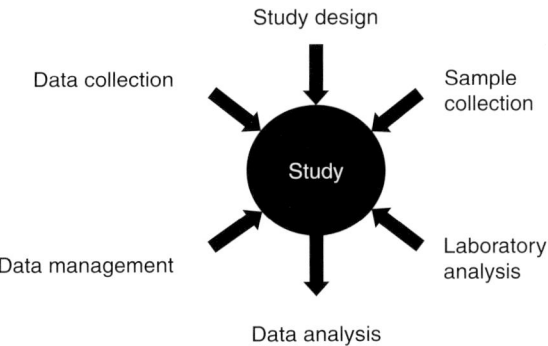

Fig. 5.1. Potential sources of error in a study.

to measure and discover. It is common for scientists to prepare a study protocol, which is a written account of the plans for the study and should include clear objectives for tackling error.

Steps two and three are to improve precision and accuracy in the study. Thomas Huxley recognized that organization is key to science: 'Science is nothing but trained and organized common sense, differing from the latter only as a veteran may differ from a raw recruit: and its methods differ from those of common sense only as far as the guardsman's cut and thrust differ from the manner in which a savage wields his club.' (Thomas H. Huxley, English biologist, 1825–1895).

The words 'precision' and 'accuracy' are often used interchangeably in lay language, but they have very specific meanings for scientists. Figure 5.2 shows an imaginary circle that represents a target and the small black dots represent bullet marks. This is analogous to a measurement made by an epidemiologist, where the cross-hairs in the centre of the target represent the truth. Of course, when measurements are made, the true value is not known, and will never be known.

A precise measurement can still be inaccurate, and vice versa. Precision is a lack of random error, where random error can be defined as 'chance'; this is variation we cannot predict. Improving precision will help to deal with one source of error and bias. The major determinant of the precision of a study is the size of the sample used. Increasing the number of people in a sample will increase the precision of the measurements. You can imagine that this may still result in inaccurate measurements overall.

A further improvement may be made through improvements in the efficiency of a study, for example by collecting a spread of outcomes, exposures, effect modifiers and confounders that is more appropriate. The spread will differ depending on the study design and context, but, broadly speaking, a sufficient number of people with the outcome, and a sufficient number of people exposed and unexposed is necessary.

Accuracy is the lack of systematic error, and when used in relation to testing it is also known as 'validity'. A measurement may have internal and external validity. Internal validity is where the measurements relate to the truth within the series of measures you make. For example, you may be making measurements of a series of weights, and the scales you use are not accurate in relation to their true mass. However, as long as the same scales are used these may possess internal validity.

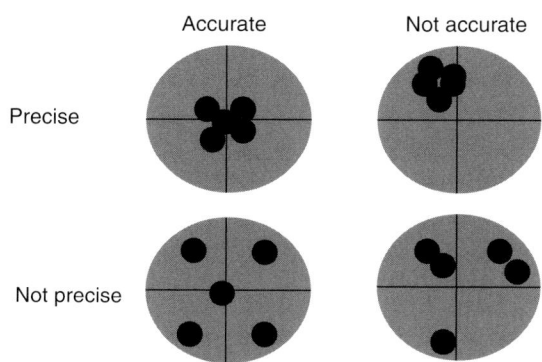

Fig. 5.2. Contrasting accuracy and precision.

External validity is where not only do the measures represent the internal relationships, but they also are accurate for external studies. Continuing the weight measurements example, if the scales are also accurate in relation to other scales then the weights are externally valid.

Bias means leaning to one side

The term 'bias', in its general usage, means to be inclined to one side with implications for influence and associated with prejudice. Bias is important for epidemiological studies as the wrong answer and inference may be obtained from a biased study. Figure 5.3a is an analogy for bias, where the tower at Pisa is supposed to be standing vertically. It has slipped to one side, and yet even this has been useful if we are to believe the apocryphal tale that Galileo Galilei dropped two cannon balls of different masses from the tower to demonstrate that their mass did not control their rate of descent.

Your role, as an epidemiologist, is to remove or reduce bias; with Fig. 5.3b a tongue-in-cheek representation of the epidemiologist's job.

The hunt for forms of bias begins with your perspective. From one angle (Fig. 5.3c) the Leaning Tower of Pisa does not lean. This is analogous to an epidemiologist looking at their study. They may think that their study contains no bias. But someone, looking from a different angle, looking at the study design and conduct differently may decide that the study does contain bias.

Three types of bias: information, selection and confounding

There are three main forms of bias: information, selection and confounding. Bias due to errors in the measurement of the information that is collected is classified as information bias; there are many forms and many are avoidable. Selection bias often occurs earlier in a study when the wrong people or subjects are chosen or recruited to a study. It is difficult to avoid and to compensate for selection bias, and to compound this situation it may often go unrecognized in a study. Bias due to confounding is a contentious issue: a confounder must first be identified and these are sometimes mixed up with other forms of bias or identified mistakenly altogether.

Selection bias: collecting the right data on the wrong people

Sampling error is one of the most important, and well understood, forms of error in an epidemiological study. Statistical teaching revolves around the creation of an understanding of this error, in the form of confidence intervals, for example. In all situations, sampling error may exist and you will be able to use simple techniques to inform you of how sampling error affects your inference.

Sources of selection bias include inappropriate selection of study subjects from the population, non-random assignment of exposure status, and the omission from the study of subjects from the analysis. Inappropriate selection involves the non-random selection of subjects from the population, selection of subjects from different or ill-defined study populations, failure to locate people to participate or loss of persons from the study population because of a health outcome under study, for example selective survival. Non-random allocation methods, for example self-selection or allocation by a clinician, can create bias. Selection bias may also occur through omission of subjects due to high losses-to-follow-up.

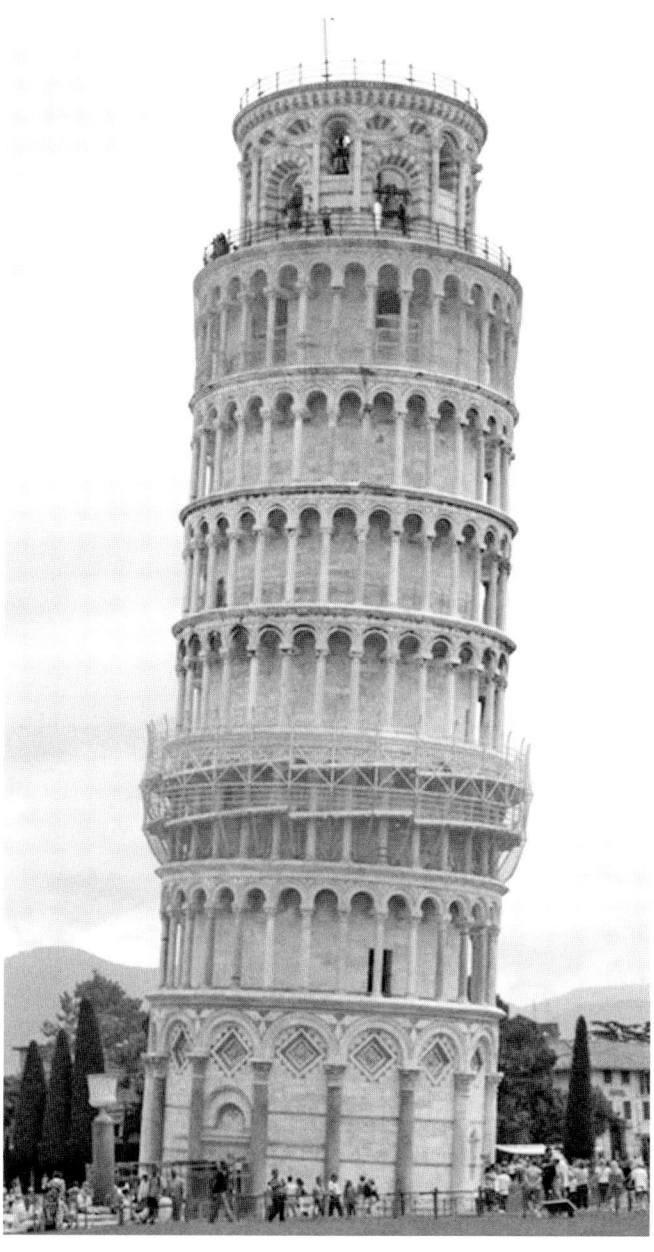

Fig. 5.3. (a) Bias is leaning to one side (the Leaning Tower of Pisa). (b) The removal of bias is an epidemiologist's job. (c) Bias also depends on your perspective.

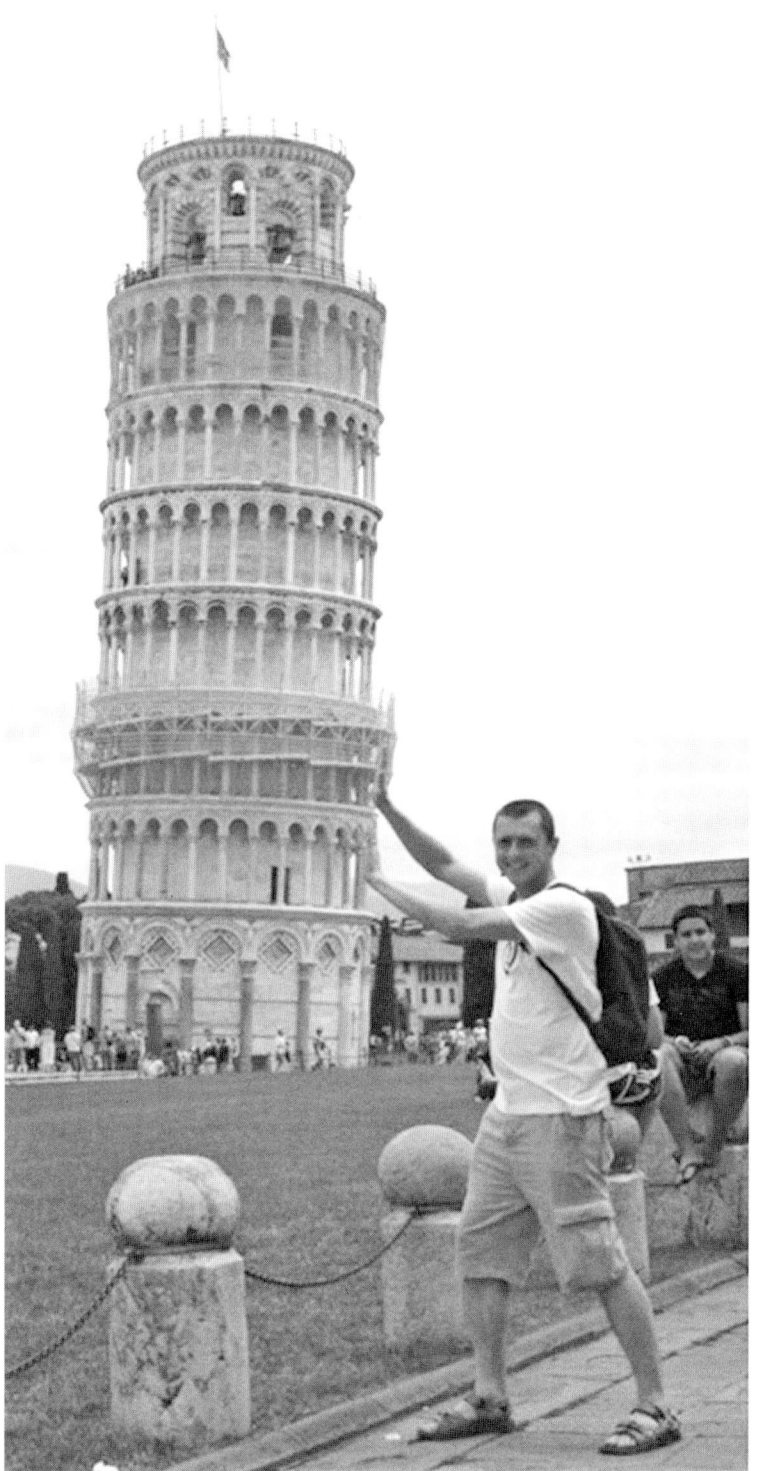

Fig. 5.3. Continued.

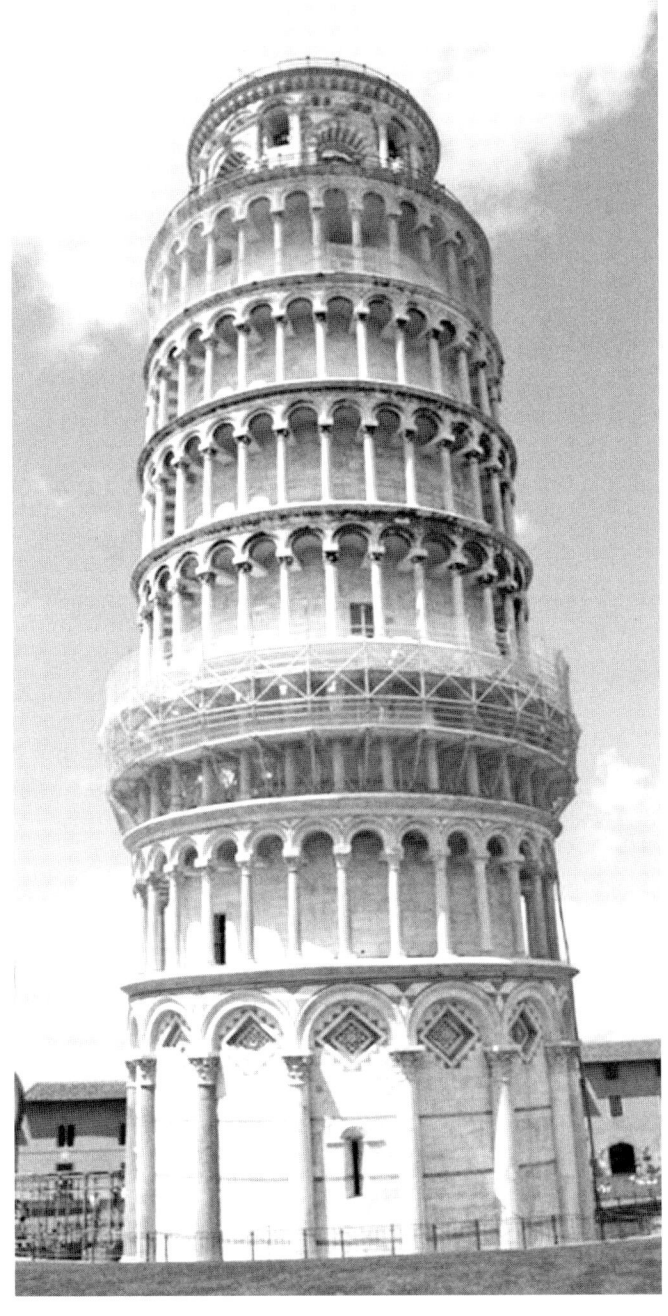

Fig. 5.3. Continued.

We can minimize selection bias when selecting study subjects by clearly defining the study population in time and place. Similarly, using sampling techniques that result in choosing groups, such as cases and controls, from the same population and using methods that result in high recruitment rates can minimize bias. Random allocation results in less bias in the assignment of exposure status in experimental studies. When study subjects are omitted from analysis there are methods to minimize loss-to-follow-up, for example follow-up phone calls, while a review of non-respondents can also provide insights and minimize bias.

Information bias: collecting the wrong data on the right people

Sources of information bias can include error within the reports from an individual, for example poor recall of past exposures. Instrument error can involve the equipment not being properly calibrated, and observer error where the researcher incorrectly uses an instrument or recording. We can minimize measurement bias by using validated and reliable tools to measure study subjects. We can train staff and monitor their use of research tools, regularly conducting quality checks of research tools used, or blinding of the study subjects and assessors to the outcomes.

Confounding: a difficult and contentious issue

Confounding, as the name suggests, involves a bewildering state of affairs. A variable is a confounder if:

1. It is an independent risk factor, a cause, of the disease.
2. It is non-randomly distributed among the exposed and non-exposed subjects.
3. It is not on the causal pathway between exposure and disease.

A confounder results in a difference between a study exposure, for example living under power lines, and a disease, for example leukaemia. This is interesting in terms of house planning, property values and compensation, amongst other things. However the missing piece of the puzzle could be a confounder, such as socio-economic status. The confounder is associated with both the study exposure and the disease you are investigating and although generates a statistically significant result for us at the end, breaks down the causal link between exposure (power lines) and disease (leukaemia).

There are many opportunities for controlling confounders. At the design phase we can ensure that confounders are not unevenly distributed among the exposed and unexposed. We can restrict those people eligible for the study by limiting the study to people with one level of a potential confounder. Stratified allocation within strata of the confounder can also reduce the risk of confounding. Matching patients in cohort studies and case-control studies also limits confounding, whilst randomization provides a method for dealing with both known and unknown confounders in experimental studies. At the analysis phase we can control for confounders demonstrating comparability between exposed and unexposed.

Summary

The acceptance of different perspectives may encourage a scientist to question openly a colleague or reputed scientist (see Box 5.2). This may seem difficult, possibly causing embarrassment or discomfort, but it is an essential part of the scientific method: the attempts to falsify existing hypotheses.

Epidemiology is about the accurate and precise estimation of a value we are looking to measure. We make observations and need to ensure these are as close as possible to the truth in order to determine cause. The process of observing can contain systematic or random errors. Epidemiologists recognize this and attempt to remove bias from research studies, identifying bias due to selection, information and confounding.

Self-test questions

Q 5.1.1: What are the three main types of bias?

Q 5.1.2: Selection bias is:
A Recording the wrong information on the right people
B Recording the right information on the wrong people
C A mixing of effects with another variable

Q 5.1.3: True or False? A confounder is a cause of the outcome and a cause of the exposure.

Q 5.1.4: Accuracy is:
A A lack of systematic error
B A lack of random error

5.2   Information Bias

- Pre-requisite sections: 5.1.
- Learning outcome: By the end of this section you should be able to explain what information bias is and how it happens.

Box 5.3 features a scene from the hit British comedy *Yes, Prime Minister*, in which the private secretary is shown how the questions asked in a survey can lead the interviewee to an answer. This is a form of information bias where the same person gives different responses to a question because they are influenced by other factors or events.

Box 5.3. 'A perfect balanced sample'

The following is an excerpt from British sitcom *Yes, Prime Minister*, first aired in 1986. The British Prime Minister's private secretary, Bernard Woolley, is speaking with Sir Humphrey, the permanent secretary, about responses to an opinion poll:

Bernard Woolley: 'The Party have had an opinion poll done and it seems all the voters are in favour of bringing back National Service.'
Sir Humphrey: 'Well, have another opinion poll done to show that they're against bringing back National Service.'
BW: 'They can't be for and against …'
SH: 'Of course they can, Bernard! Have you ever been surveyed?'

Sir Humphrey demonstrates:

SH: 'Mr. Woolley, are you worried about the number of young people without jobs?'
BW: 'Yes'
SH: 'Are you worried about the rise in crime among teenagers?'
BW: 'Yes'
SH: 'Do you think there is a lack of discipline in our Comprehensive schools?'
BW: 'Yes'
SH: 'Do you think young people welcome some authority and leadership in their lives?'
BW: 'Yes'
SH: 'Do you think they respond to a challenge?'
BW: 'Yes'
SH: 'Would you be in favour of reintroducing National Service?'
BW: 'Oh … well, I suppose I might be.'
SH: 'Yes or no?'
BW: 'Yes'

Sir Humphrey now takes the opposite approach:

SH: 'Mr. Woolley, are you worried about the danger of war?'
BW: 'Yes'
SH: 'Are you worried about the growth of armaments?'
BW: 'Yes'
SH: 'Do you think there is a danger in giving young people guns and teaching them how to kill?'
BW: 'Yes'
SH: 'Do you think it is wrong to force people to take up arms against their will?'
BW: 'Yes'
SH: 'Would you oppose the reintroduction of National Service?'
BW: 'Yes'
SH: 'There you are, you see, Bernard? The perfect balanced sample.'

In this way Sir Humphrey has led Bernard into answering both 'yes' and 'no' to the same question. This is a form of information bias: the same person gives different responses due to other influences.

Reproduced from *Yes, Prime Minister*, by Jonathan Lynn and Antony Jay with permission from the authors. © Jonathan Lynn and Antony Jay.

Bias from collecting the wrong data on the right people

Researchers go to great lengths to recruit an appropriate sample from the population in which the researchers are interested. Following selection and recruitment of participants, the data must be collected in relation to the outcome, the exposure and other relevant variables. All of the hard work in recruiting people may be spoiled by collecting the wrong data where the data in some way does not represent the true data you wish to collect. This was highlighted by Sir Humphrey when the same person, in a different situation, gives opposite answers to the same question. There are a number of ways information bias may occur and it may happen in all types of study design.

Recall bias relates to prior events influencing answers

Many epidemiology studies need people to report on circumstances or events pertinent to the hypothesis under investigation, known as 'recall'. The respondent's recall will be affected by their recollection of the event and other external pressures.

Recall may be biased accidentally or sometimes intentionally by the respondent. An example of intentionally biased recall occurs in nutrition research where it is common for a person to underestimate their alcohol intake. Another form of recall bias comes about when study subjects give answers they feel they should give, due to pressure from peers, or society. Box 5.4 gives an example of recall bias when people are asked about the coffee they like to drink. Many people will state what they feel they should like, the type of coffee perceived as the best. However in truth most people prefer a different sort of coffee.

A medical example may help to reinforce this. Imagine a case-control study of a serious childhood disease, such as diabetes, where the scientist wishes to find out about breastfeeding of the child. When questioned, the parents of control children who do not have diabetes will likely respond without prejudice – their child does not have the serious illness under investigation, and they feel no guilt. It is perfectly understandable that a parent with an unwell child has spent time reflecting on important events in the child's life, and will, when asked, respond differently to the same person if in a counterfactual world they had a healthy child. This may be conscious or unconscious, but either way may change their recall of these events, leading to recall bias.

Box 5.4. How do you like your coffee?

Malcolm Gladwell recounts a story about an expert in taste, Howard Moskowitz, who researched coffee extensively. If asked, 'What sort of coffee do you like?' a lot of people reply along the lines of 'a dark, rich, hearty roast'. According to Moskowitz, however, most people in practice prefer 'milky, weak coffee', a result revealed through taste tests. People may answer a question to the best of their ability but not accurately describe their true preference (Gladwell, 2004).

Gladwell, M. (2004, February) Malcolm Gladwell on spaghetti sauce [Video file]. Retrieved from http://www.ted.com/talks/malcolm_gladwell_on_spaghetti_sauce.html (accessed 30 September 2012).

Questions should be carefully designed

As Sir Humphrey demonstrated in Box 5.3, the form of the questions given to a study subject may influence the recall of events. There has been a great deal of work in how best to design questions and questionnaires. It may seem that one of the easiest ways to avoid bias is to request answers with a quantitative response. For example, you may ask how many weeks gestation a baby was when born. This may seem a quantitative, objective measure. But this may lead to answers that are perceived as a 'normal' length of pregnancy, such as 40 weeks.

Questionnaires should be designed to not lead a participant into a certain answer. Sir Humphrey did this very well: his approach was to lead Bernard to begin to think about the young people in the country, asking if there was a lack of discipline among teenagers. This led to his perception of the importance of authority and leadership and eventually to asking about the reintroduction of National Service, to which Bernard answered 'Yes'. Immediately after this exchange Sir Humphrey asked if teaching teenagers to use guns was dangerous, and forcing guns on people was wrong. When asked the same question about National Service he responded 'No'.

Respondents might also give incorrect answers to impress the interviewer. This type of error is the most difficult to prevent because it results from deceit on the part of the responder. Knowing why a study is being conducted may create incorrect responses. A classic example is the question: What is your income? If a government agency is asking, a different figure may be provided than the respondent would give on an application for a home mortgage. One way to guard against such bias is to camouflage the study's goals; another remedy is to make the questions very specific, allowing no room for personal interpretation. For example, 'Where are you employed?' could be followed by 'What is your salary?' and 'Do you have any extra jobs?' A sequence of such questions may produce more accurate information.

Interviewers must be trained and monitored

When a study uses people employed as interviewers, the epidemiologists must be very careful to avoid bias introduced by their actions, known as 'interviewer bias'. It is common for healthcare professionals, such as nurses, to be employed as interviewers on studies; these people have been trained to assess patients, to find out information, to take histories. This style, while appropriate for clinical care, is often not appropriate for a scientific study. These skills may not be helpful when asking structured questions for a study in epidemiology.

Interviewers must be trained in the specific questionnaire being used, and monitored as closely as possible, which may include making recordings that can be listened to by a trainer afterwards to pick up any areas where the interviewer is leading the respondent. No two interviewers are alike and the same person may provide different answers to different interviewers.

Questions should be clear, be non-offensive and enable the respondent to answer correctly. The interviewers should avoid leading questions, or the use of language that may lead the respondent to answering in a certain way. Using terms such as 'normal', or 'standard' may make the respondent concerned that their response will not be correct as it is not 'standard'.

Interviewers should not know the disease status of the participants

A further complication, particularly for retrospective studies where a diagnosis has already been made, comes about when the interviewer knows the disease status of the respondent. For example, a healthcare professional, knowing that a person has a serious disease, may unconsciously lead the questions so that the respondent's answers fit what the interviewer feels will be appropriate. Under these circumstances it is best if the interviewer is blinded to the status of a person they are interviewing.

This is not always possible or ethical, in that the respondent may have clear signs of the disease under study, or it may be felt that the interviewer needs to know about any serious health issues that may have a bearing on the interview. This may include appropriate changes to the length of the interview, giving breaks during the interview, or the location of the interview.

Surrogate sources of data may be useful but should be carefully examined

It is feasible that a study participant may not be able to volunteer the data that is required. Many participants may be too young to answer, or language difficulties may interfere. It is also possible a person may be too unwell to respond, or find it too difficult emotionally. In these situations it is common for epidemiologists to seek answers from surrogates. These may be family or friends who are close to the subject and it is hoped will provide accurate information.

Information from surrogates should be carefully collected. A surrogate may not know about personal habits or illegal practices, such as recreational drug use. They may also wish to avoid implied criticism, leading to responses that are not as accurate as they may be when obtained directly from the participant.

Bias may occur where a diagnosis has implications

In clinical practice, in order to reinforce a diagnosis, it is possible that the clinical diagnosis may drive information collected. This may be due to legal, financial or societal pressures. There are many examples, and it is not possible to give a simple formula to identify this happening. It is up to the epidemiologist to understand the situation and think carefully.

For example, a diagnosis of malignant mesothelioma, a rare form of cancer of the lung that is strongly associated with exposure to asbestos, may lead to the assignment of the sufferer to an occupation with asbestos exposure. However, in the general population, where a person has not been diagnosed with mesothelioma, it is less likely a person will be categorized as exposed to asbestos. This may be an underestimate of true exposure in those without that diagnosis.

Misclassification bias occurs when data is incorrectly categorized

Even when correct data has been collected, the scientists may create bias through analytical practices. An analyst may place data into categories, which is a common practice, and these categories may relate to the outcome, exposure or other variables. The analyst must avoid placing the response into the wrong category.

There are two forms of misclassification. Non-differential misclassification is not related to any important variable. An example of this is where there is no difference in classification between cases and non-cases in a case-control study, but there is still some misclassification, for example an under-estimate of fat intake in both diabetic and non-diabetic subjects. There is a common misconception that this always leads the estimates of risk to be biased towards null. For this reason it is often seen as acceptable, but this may lead to false comfort.

Differential misclassification is where the placement of data into categories is different between important groups in the study. For example, in a case-control study, information may be classified differently between cases and controls. An example of this is in studies of inflammation of the stomach lining, known as gastritis. This is often caused by a pathogen known as *Helicobacter pylori*, knowledge which may lead a pathologist assessing biopsies for evidence of infection to classify people with gastritis as having *H. pylori* infection in the presence of gastritis. This leads to a potential for substantial differential misclassification.

Medical records may reduce recall bias

Abstractions from medical records are often used in epidemiologic studies. They are seen as an objective set of information, unlikely to be affected by recall or misclassification. However, careful consideration should be given to the quality of the data because medical data is recorded for diagnostic and treatment purposes, not for research.

For example, data are usually more complete when a clear diagnosis has been established, as many records will be a report of the symptoms and signs, and not a clinical diagnosis. Better quality diagnosis is usually achieved in patients with severe disease.

Life events may help to improve recall

A method that has been used by some studies is to link the recall of events with major external or life events. If you were an adult in 1963, and I asked you where you were on a random date, such as 22nd of November, it is unlikely you will remember. However, if I asked you where you were when you heard about John F. Kennedy being assassinated, on 22nd November 1963, it is much more likely you remember.

This way to help respondents to remember some of their behaviour from a period of time ago uses major life events as emotional and memory triggers. For example, it may be possible to use events in a person's life such as births, deaths or marriages to aid memory recall. Derren Brown, a famous British illusionist, mentalist and sceptic, in his book *Tricks of the Mind*, describes how memory recall is more easily achieved when a link between an emotion and the thing to remember is made (Brown, 2007).

Summary

Information is key to the study of epidemiology. The epidemiologist may have spent considerable effort in selecting the most appropriate study subjects in their sample. The data, or information, must then be collected to avoid biases. Commonly seen bias includes that from interviewers and inappropriate questions. Other sources of data, such as surrogates and medical records, may be used but these must also be treated with caution. Bias due to recall may be avoided with some exploitation of human nature and the ability of the mind to recall events when linked with other life events.

Self-test questions

Q 5.2.1: Bias in epidemiological studies:
A Cannot be anticipated at the study-design stage
B Leads to random error due to confounding
C May arise because of selection of cases

Q 5.2.2: A cohort study gathers data about each participant through an interview with an interviewer. The interviewer has ten questions to ask the participants and is free to word the questions in the way he/she feels is best understood by the participant. This style of interview would lead to which form of bias?
A Selection bias
B Information bias
C Confounding bias

Q 5.2.3: Information bias in epidemiological studies:
A Can be anticipated at the study-design stage
B May arise because of selection of cases
C Seldom distorts effect estimates

5.3 Selection Bias

- Pre-requisite sections: 5.1.
- Learning outcome: By the end of this section you should be able to explain what selection bias is and how it happens.

All epidemiological studies, whether experimental or observational in nature, are prone to various errors that can lead to bias. One of these, known as selection bias, is where an error in choosing the participants occurs. The resultant biases may prove catastrophic to a study. Any study that has a biased selection of participants may already have determined the results that will be obtained through an artefact of the recruitment process.

The population must first be defined

When an epidemiologist conducts a research study one of the first tasks is to define the population and create a sample to study. The sampling frame must reflect the epidemiological triad of time, place and person, by incorporating the geographical, temporal and other demographic aspects to create the population from which a sample is to be taken.

The population definition may be biased at this point. For example, the unusually named 'length time bias' comes about when a researcher chooses temporal restrictions to a study that may influence the results. A temporal trend can be made to look different by changing the start and end points. Figure 5.4 shows a simple illustration of this where a study looks at the incidence of a disease over time. The top plot shows a total of 20 years of data, and there is evidence of increases and decreases, leading to the conclusion of a fairly level incidence overall. The second and third plots show two 'slices' of the time, and very different conclusions would be found for the different slices. In the same way, trials may be terminated early, for ethical or other reasons, but this may lead to the wrong conclusion being drawn.

The epidemiologist, once a population has been defined, must identify all members of a population which is to be sampled. This is not a straightforward task, most societies have hidden structures, for example people may be in difficult-to-reach parts of society: they may be homeless or not registered with a healthcare practitioner. This leads to a situation where there is an 'ignored' section of the population. This often forms the most difficult group of people to sample.

A random sampling strategy is best

There are many methods employed by epidemiologists to sample people. Random selection is always preferred where possible, though this may not be achievable.

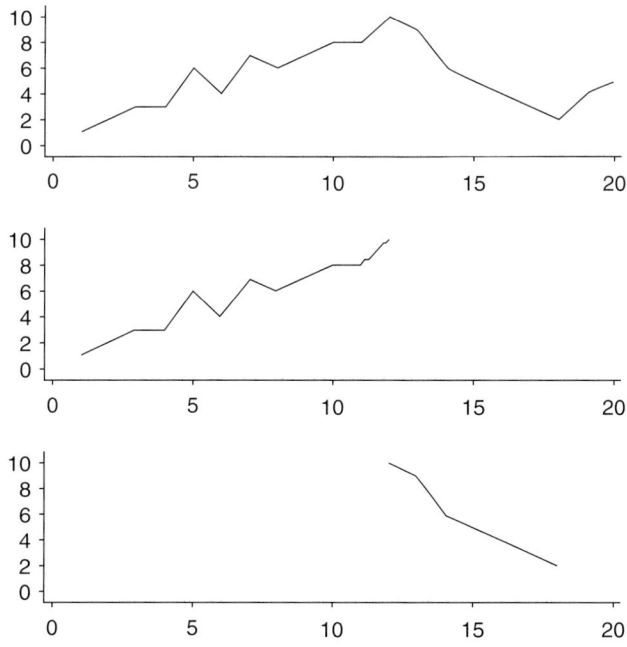

Fig. 5.4. A study of incidence over time.

Random selection from lists, for people with a disease of interest, or for those without a disease, is usually implemented in research studies. In some countries, such as in the United Kingdom, community doctors maintain lists of patients which can be used to sample from. Even these lists may not contain members of an ignored population, such as people in lower socio-economic status groups, or people who exclusively use private medicine.

Most countries in the world maintain registers of births and deaths. These may be used as a convenient sampling frame, particularly for birth cohorts. Particularly popular in the USA is the use of random digit telephone dialling, where an organization is employed to contact potential study subjects by telephone. Random digit dialling will only manage to contact people who own a telephone and who are in their house at the time the phone call is made.

Healthy worker effect should be identified

A sampling frame may contain hidden structure that is unwanted for a particular study. The 'healthy worker effect' occurs where sampling of individuals takes place to selectively include or exclude individuals who are making a living from employment. People who work are, on average, healthier than people who do not work, which may be because people who are not working are unable to work due to illness, or it may be because the act of working imparts some health benefits.

An example of a healthy worker effect could be seen if an occupational setting was used to recruit individuals for a study. These people will be on average healthier overall than the general population. The opposite effect may be seen when individuals are recruited from a shopping mall during a working day hence weighting recruitment towards non-workers. The epidemiologist must be aware of this possibility when designing a sampling frame.

Participants may self-select or refuse

Voluntary participation in health-related studies is rarely 100%, and there is evidence it has been declining over time (Hartge, 1999). Any study requiring a personal questionnaire, biometric measurements, access to medical records or biological samples is hampered by participation. A particular problem for epidemiological research arises when participation is different between study groups, such as cases and controls, or treatment and control groups. Unfortunately, whether or not an individual agrees to participate in a project is often associated with the health outcome and exposure under investigation; this may lead to biased estimates of risk (Rothman and Greenland, 1998).

It is not uncommon for people to contact a study organizer requesting to be involved in a particular study. Involvement of such participants should be carefully judged because they may have some particular connection to an environmental or genetic component of a disease and therefore do not truly represent the study population.

Attrition bias is a kind of selection bias caused by the loss of participants from a study or trial. Loss may be due to the participants actively dropping out, or passively not responding to requests to participate. It is particularly problematic when attrition is unequal with regard to exposure or outcome.

Differential participation between important study subgroups may arise in commonly used study designs such as the case-control study. Frequently, problems may arise when the design of the study is retrospective to the development of the disease of interest. This leads to differing motivation amongst potential participants, and often different sampling frames being used to capture the various categories of participant.

As Schlesselman stated in his book about case-control studies (Schlesselman and Stolley, 1982): 'The best designed sampling scheme … can be vitiated by high rates of refusal'. The case-control study has become embedded as a standard epidemiological tool, with application to a wide range of human disease research. The inherent strength of this design, that it uses individual rather than aggregated data, is also a potential weakness.

Exploring non-participation is difficult

Many studies are unable to assess the characteristics of those individuals that did not participate, leading to an absence of information about the magnitude of participation bias and its potential impact. Exploring non-participants has relied on re-approaching non-participants and asking a restricted number of questions. However, even when the identities of non-participants are known, practical and ethical considerations often prohibit the use of such methods.

Some studies, for example the United Kingdom Childhood Cancer Study, provided a valuable opportunity to investigate the potential impact of participation (UKCCS Investigators, 2000). It was argued that most of the cases arising in the target population were recruited: multiple sources of case notification were interrogated. The initial selection of control children has been shown to be reassuringly similar to the target population it was designed to represent (Law *et al.*, 2002). In contrast, it has been demonstrated that control participation was associated with a measure of socio-economic status, where it is thought that this acts as a proxy for closely related factors, such as educational status, which directly influences willingness to participate in the study as a control.

Suggested solutions to selection bias

A large number of possible solutions to selection bias have been suggested. This follows the important step of recognizing that selection bias may be a problem. When using most study designs, researchers are governed by practical and ethical constraints which require individuals to agree to participate. Of course, the best and most reliable option is to avoid the problem in the first place. When a study can be conducted without requiring active participation from study subjects the design may allow a selection bias-free implementation. However, as most studies do require permission from study subjects, they are left open to error in selection and its effects.

First choice controls, those identified first regardless of their choice to participate or not, have been used. For example, Law and colleagues used all first choice controls without requiring their participation (Law *et al.*, 2003). This is because the exposure measures were derived from postal addresses linked to national census data. These controls should be a representative sample of the target population, given the initial selection procedures are robust.

Another approach to dealing with selection bias is to 'adjust' for variables thought to cause, or influence, selection in a statistical model. Some authors have argued that adjusting for selection bias is identical to the process of adjusting for confounding: the variables associated with selection are incorporated into a regression model (e.g. Breslow and Day, 1980). However, when the variable is not a confounder in this context (McNamee, 2003), there is no meaningful way to 'adjust' for its complex influence on the outcome. When it is a true confounder, the conclusion is quite different: statistical adjustment by inclusion of the variable in the model recovers accurately and consistently the population relative risk.

In contrast to the case-control study, the cohort study design has fewer problems with recruitment and participation being differential between groups. Historical cohorts may sometimes require participants to volunteer after the disease outcome is known, and so be more prone to the problem than traditional cohorts, but such historical or 'retrospective' cohorts are less common than their traditional counterparts (Henderson and Page, 2007).

The randomized controlled trial uses an analysis method known as the 'intention to treat', where initial assignments to either active or control groups are analysed. This is despite the fact that some studies have high levels of drop out, for example where a treatment is particularly uncomfortable or unsuccessful.

Summary

Selection bias, choosing the wrong people, is an important bias for epidemiological studies. There are many types, some of the most common being bias due to differential participation and the healthy worker effect. As with all bias, avoiding it in the first place is the best approach. But, this is not always practical, or ethical. Some studies will inevitably suffer from participation bias. The onus is on the researcher to explore the causes of the bias, and try to estimate how this will impact on the inference and results.

Self-test questions

Q 5.3.1: In an experiment to compare two treatments, subjects are allocated at random so that:
A The experimenter will not know which treatment the subjects receive
B The sample may be compared to a known population
C The two groups will be as similar as possible, apart from treatment
D Treatments may be assigned according to the characteristics of the subject

Q 5.3.2: True or false? Differential participation between cases and controls is a form of selection bias.

Q 5.3.3: Selection bias is:
A Collecting the wrong data on the right people.
B Collecting the right data on the wrong people.

Q 5.3.4: Recruiting participants from an occupational setting runs the risk of:
A The healthy worker effect
B Loss-to-follow-up
C Participation bias

Q 5.3.5: Which sampling strategies minimize selection bias?
A Random digit dialling
B Snowballing
C Disease register
D Electoral roll

5.4 Confounding

● Pre-requisite sections: 2.2, 2.3, 5.1.
● Learning outcome: By the end of this section you should be able to describe confounding and ways to identify a confounder.

Confounding, and the bias a confounder can induce, is a major problem for epidemiology, and it is unfortunately fairly common. Confounding can generate biased results when examining the association between an exposure and an outcome. As Pearl (Pearl, 2000) stated: 'Confounding represents one of the most fundamental impediments to the elucidation of causal inferences from empirical data'. Despite this, there is debate about the definition and identification of a confounder: it is a complex issue.

A definition of a confounder

The definitions of confounding, and there are many versions, may be divided broadly into two main types: comparability-based and collapsibility-based (Greenland and Robins, 1986). In the comparability-based definition, confounding is said to occur when there are differences in outcome in the unexposed and exposed populations that are not due to the exposure, but are due to other variables that may be referred to as confounders. The collapsibility-based definition reflects the view that confounding may be reduced or eliminated through statistical adjustment. The second type of definition is less useful for understanding the process, as focusing on confounding as a causal rather than a statistical issue leads one to adopt the comparability-based definition.

There are three conditions that must be satisfied for a variable to be considered a confounder:

1. The confounder variable must cause or prevent the outcome you are investigating, or be a proxy for the cause.
2. A confounder is a variable that is correlated with the putative causative variable, or exposure, that you are investigating.

3. The confounder variable must not be an effect or consequence of the exposure: it is not on the causal pathway.

It is because of these associations that a simple statistical analysis between the putative exposure and outcome will lead to a potentially incorrect interpretation. Your analyses will be biased, or you will not be able to be certain that your results are not biased. Either way, it spells trouble for the analysis.

A simple example illustrates confounding

Let's use an unlikely example to illustrate these difficulties. Imagine there was a case-control study of lung cancer, with cases being people with lung cancer and controls people without lung cancer. An epidemiologist examined the fingers of the participants and discovered that those people with yellow-stained fingers had a higher risk of lung cancer compared to those without yellow-stained fingers. Is this a true effect? Do we really think that yellow staining on fingers is a cause of lung cancer?

Of course not. With hindsight we know this is probably due to another factor: cigarette smoking. Should we consider cigarette smoking to be a true confounder in this example? We step through the three conditions for cigarette smoking to be considered a confounder for yellow-stained fingers causing lung cancer:

1. Cigarette smoking, the potential confounder, is a cause of lung cancer, the outcome. Condition 1 is satisfied.
2. Cigarette smoking is correlated with yellow fingers, the putative exposure. Indeed smoking actually caused the stains. Condition 2 is satisfied.
3. Smoking is not caused by the exposure under study, yellow-stained fingers. This means that yellow-stained fingers are not on the causal pathway. Condition 3 is satisfied.

Smoking is therefore a confounder and it is important to recognize smoking as a confounder, as the inference that yellow-stained fingers cause lung cancer is not correct. This is a very simple example, and it is rare for the solution to be so obvious.

There is no objective method to identify a confounder

An epidemiologist, when faced with a new study or the data from an existing study, must be able to identify confounders; many studies will have more than one confounder. How does an epidemiologist identify that a confounder is operating?

The epidemiologist may look at their data and discover statistical associations. For example, she may discover that an exposure is correlated with another variable. However, the identification of confounding should not be solely based on a study sample, apparent confounding may be present in a study due to sampling and not true confounding in the population. The epidemiologist should use a consensus of opinion to help inform the decision.

Returning to the example, we made a decision that yellow-stained fingers was due to cigarette smoking. This is a consensus opinion, and does not need to be present within the study sample. When the epidemiologist looks at her data she may find that there are many other associations between the exposure and potential confounding variables. There is no objective test that can be applied to decide on the status of a variable as a confounder. This often leads to researchers putting many variables as confounders.

If you take a look at the research articles in many medical journals, you will see listed in the tables words such as 'adjusted for ...'. This is where the analyst has decided that there are potential confounders and these should be adjusted in the model. It is often not clear why these were chosen, nor the impact they will have on the analysis through using them as an adjustment.

Use causal diagrams to identify confounding

Causal diagrams, in the form of directed acyclic graphs (DAGs) may be used to define and identify variables thought to act as potential confounders. The DAG allows the epidemiologist to develop a visual summary of the likely and speculative causal links between exposures, outcome and possible confounders. DAGs have become increasingly popular in epidemiology for modelling cause and effect and they offer a systematic and objective approach to identify confounders.

These diagrams are constructed using prior knowledge and, in the case of speculative and hypothesized relationships, on conjecture. Potential confounding variables can be placed into the DAG, with all of the appropriate causal relationships specified. To determine if confounding is present the following algorithm is applied to the DAG (Greenland *et al.*, 1999):

1. Delete all arrows that exit from the exposure variable. This is equivalent to removing all effects that the exposure may have on other variables.
2. Check if there is an unblocked path from exposure to outcome. This is known as a 'backdoor path', and is equivalent to examining whether exposure and outcome have a common cause. A backdoor path is where one exits a node along an arc pointing into it, against the causal direction, to another node across any number of arcs pointing in either direction. A path is blocked when there is a 'collider' on the path (see Section 2.3 for a definition). A node becomes a collider where both arcs of the path entering and leaving the node have arrows pointing into it.
3. If there are no unblocked backdoor paths the relationship between exposure and outcome should not be subject to potential confounding from the variables included in the DAG.

Returning to our simple example, Fig. 5.5 shows a DAG constructed looking at stained fingers (E), cigarette smoking (A) and the outcome which is lung cancer (O).

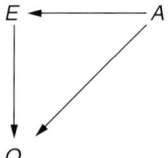

Fig. 5.5. Directed acyclic graph for the yellow-stained finger and lung cancer project. Key to variables: E – exposure (yellow-stained fingers), O – outcome (lung cancer), A – additional (cigarette smoking).

Using the algorithm above, we may remove the arrow from E to O. There is a backdoor path from E to O via the A, cigarette smoking. Therefore the variable A, cigarette smoking, should be considered a confounder.

Let's now examine a more complex example. In order to check if the relationship of exposure on the outcome in Fig. 5.6 is subject to potential confounding, we may use the same algorithm as introduced above. When the arrow is deleted, it leaves three unblocked backdoor paths from exposure to outcome:

E →C →O
E →A →C →O
E →C →B →O

From this exercise we can infer that the variables A, B and C in some way may be considered confounders on the exposure to outcome causal pathway.

How to deal with confounding

Dealing with confounding bias is essential to ensure that the results and interpretation of a study are appropriate. There are two main ways to do this: before the analysis phase and during the analysis phase. Before the analysis the design may avoid bias. The randomized controlled trial is designed to avoid confounding; participants are randomized to exposure groups, thus leaving no association between exposure and potential confounders. This happens in a successfully randomized RCT where potential confounding variables are balanced between groups. This is also important when there are both measured and unmeasured confounders. It is feasible that a researcher will not be aware of some potential confounders, and the randomization process should alleviate their effects also.

Randomization does not take place in an observational study design, but other methods may be used. In a case-control study, matching of controls to cases on the basis of confounder variables is used. For example, if the researcher decides that age and sex are potential confounders then the controls may be selected to match the profile of the cases' age and sex. This does not, however, deal with unmeasured confounders. It also restricts the analysis: the scientist is not able to examine the impact of the confounding variables on the risk of disease.

The confounder may also be dealt with during the analysis of the data. It is common for observational studies to contain at least one confounder that the study is unable to eliminate through manipulation of the design. It is then left to

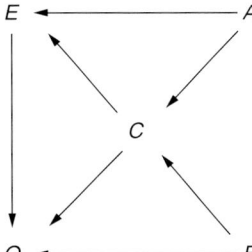

Fig. 5.6. Hypothetical directed acyclic graph. Key to variables: E – exposure, O – outcome, A, B, C – additional variables.

the scientist to analyse the study to take account of the confounder. One way to do this is to analyse the subgroups of the confounder separately. In this way the analyst should be able to construct homogeneous categories of the confounder and these stratum-specific estimates may then be combined into an overall estimate of the risk of the disease in relation to the exposure. A more standard approach with the advent of statistical computer packages is to enter the confounder into a statistical model to adjust for its effects. Both of these methods produce estimates of risk that are, both in theory and practice, not affected by the confounder.

DAGs identify the effect of adjusting for a confounder

DAGs may also be used to identify the extent to which adjustment for a confounding variable creates further confounding which in turn requires adjustment (Greenland *et al.*, 1999). DAGs help define a subset of potential confounders that is a subset selected from all identified potential confounders, sufficient to adjust for confounding. Indeed, DAGs can be used to identify the full range of such subsets and thereby test and select the most appropriate one to use (Greenland *et al.*, 1999).

DAGs may also be used to determine the sufficient set of confounders. This involves examining the effect of adjusting smaller number of variables on the pathway. The analyst is looking for an adjustment to 'block' the path and no longer allow a backdoor path from exposure to outcome. There can be more than one minimally sufficient set, and these sets vary in size and may not necessarily overlap (Greenland *et al.*, 1999).

Summary

Confounding is an important issue for epidemiology. It is a mixing up of the effects of variables, where the epidemiologist may assume that the observed effects between an exposure and an outcome are clear. But a second variable, known as the confounder, may have created or otherwise impacted on, this relationship.

A good tool for exploring your study to identify confounders is the DAG. DAGs encourage researchers to formally structure presumed and predicted causal pathways. With satisfactory construction they can be used to identify sufficient sets of confounders, which will greatly help the analyst to do the analysis.

Once a sufficient set of confounders has been identified the analyst may adjust for them. This may be done by examining risks within strata of the confounders, or through incorporating the confounders into a statistical model.

Self-test questions

Q 5.4.1: True or false? A confounder must be a cause of the outcome.

Q 5.4.2: True or false? A confounder must not be associated with the exposure of interest.

Q 5.4.3: A randomized controlled trial is less likely to be affected by confounding because of:
A The control group
B The treatment group
C The random allocation to groups
D The loss-to-follow-up

Further Reading

Bernhardt, V.L. (1998) *Multiple Measures*, Invited Monograph No. 4. California Association for Supervision and Curriculum Development (CASCD).

Answers and Feedback

A 1.1.1: The epidemiological triad describes the distribution of disease by three categories, the time, the place and the person. The time can be anything from the decade or century through to a day or even seconds. The place most often refers to a geographical location, and the person refers to factors relevant to the host, such as the sex of the person or their age.

A 1.1.2: B and C are correct. An exposure and risk factors are both terms that may be used to describe a putative cause of a disease. An outcome is the thing we are trying to describe, and a cluster is a group of diseases in one location and/or time.

A 1.1.3: B is correct.

A 1.1.4: All of these were considered approaches to stopping the spread of cholera. But the most effective was to remove the water pump handle of the infected water source.

A 1.1.5: She was the first female member of the Royal Statistical Society, and later became a member of the American Statistical Association.

A 1.2.1: A is correct – scientific method dictates that a hypothesis is never conclusive. This may be unsatisfactory, and advice and interventions can proceed on the basis of existing hypotheses, even though sometimes they are shown to be incorrect and rejected.

A 1.2.2: B is correct. Using scientific method the scientist should not accept a study as true, but should continue to test the hypothesis. Of course, at some point, it is appropriate that the weight of evidence will finally convince a scientist of the truth in a hypothesis.

A 1.2.3: The null hypothesis sets out a position opposite to one we are interested in, or at least a hypothesis that describes no effect.

A 1.2.4: Validity is how close a measurement is to the truth. The truth is not something we know with certainty.

A 1.3.1: Doll and Hill designed a cohort based on British doctors. These provided a simple group to identify and follow up due to their registration with the British General Medical Council.

A 1.3.2: This must be estimated, but best estimates suggest over 6,000,000 people have been saved from premature death.

A 1.3.3: Evidence-based medicine (EBM) aims to use scientific and other forms of evidence to underpin practice. Decisions, such as diagnosis and treatment, are based on the most up-to-date information that has been determined by a body of expert opinion.

A 1.3.4: Lemon juice.

A 1.4.1: A scientist generally creates a sample, which is a restricted, smaller, version of the population. This is to allow the scientist to make an inference without the expense of looking at the whole population.

A 1.4.2: The size of the population will generally make it impossible to collect every single member of the population. The finance and time required makes this unfeasible.

A 1.4.3: Purposive and Snowball are not methods that can be classed as a random sampling method. Cluster sampling uses a random approach to sampling.

A 1.5.1: They are the development of a formal logic system and the experimental method.

A 1.5.2: The controlled experiment compares the experimental or intervention group with the control group.

A 1.5.3: A natural experiment uses a situation that has occurred that was not designed by the scientist.

A 1.5.4: An observational study will be essential when it is not feasible or ethical to conduct an experiment.

A 1.6.1: Public health initiatives (for example sewers, clean water) and economic development (for example improving nutrition).

A 1.6.2: S – Subjective: What did the patient say? O – Objective: What evidence of ill-health have I elicited? A – Assessment: What do I make of the situation? P – Plan: What am I going to do?

A 1.6.3: A temporary and sanctioned form of illness behaviour which had the benefit of giving an individual a reason for not completing their social responsibilities.

A 1.6.4: True.

A 2.1.1: Intervene on the exposure, by removing it. We may also be able to create therapies that alleviate or cure the disease.

A 2.1.2: A counterfactual is an identical situation but with one thing changed. For example, a counterfactual for a study to see whether mobile phones cause cancer, would be identical except mobile phones would not be present.

A 2.1.3: The randomized controlled trial comes closest to representing the counterfactual. In reality, none of these studies actually have a counterfactual.

A 2.1.4: The latent period of a disease is B, the time from exposure to a cause to onset of disease.

A 2.2.1: All four may be used, but in practice A, C and D are useful in the real world.

A 2.2.2: The trial is an experimental method, where one of the groups in the trial may represent the counterfactual world. It is, of course, not possible to have a counterfactual population, but the RCT is the closest you can get to one.

A 2.2.3: A is a counterfactual population, as the cases of a disease not given the new drug is a group of controls designed to represent the counterfactual population. The group given the new drug, in B, are not really representing the counterfactual population, although it could be argued that they represent the counterfactual population for the controls group not receiving the new drug. The people without the disease, in C, do not represent the counterfactual population as some of these will have been exposed, and some will not have been. This is a case-control study design. Those people in D represent a counterfactual as none of them were exposed. The assumption is that there is also a group of people without a disease at the start of the study who were exposed. This is a cohort study design.

A 2.3.1: A variable is represented as a node. An arc and line are the arrows in a DAG. The confounder is a variable, but it is a specific type of variable.

A 3.1.1: Cervical cancer incidence may have fallen for a number of reasons. The most likely explanation is the use of cervical screening that detects pre-cancerous lesions. The cause of the cancer may have been removed from the population, or the genetic profile of the population may have changed.

A 3.2.1: Anecdote, by definition, relates to an isolated event that is unpublished. Science may be able to use the anecdote to pursue a certain avenue for research, but it cannot be tested directly. The observation must be able to be falsified and the collection of the data for the anecdote will not be conducted sufficiently rigorously to meet the standards required. Anecdote also often refers to an extreme event, which may be due to chance alone.

A 3.2.2: There are many examples, but we have focused on the lower rates of cervical cancer in nuns. With hindsight this related to the sexual activity of nuns, and offered insight into the cause of the disease. The famous studies of Doll and Hill, that led to evidence that smoking tobacco causes lung cancer, were in part motivated by the concerns that tarmac from road-building was causing the disease. This is an anecdote that was shown to be incorrect, but did lead to an important discovery.

A 3.2.3: This is not true. It is possible that some anecdotes may be able to be tested. The key is whether the observation was done fairly and the result can be tested which can give the result of either a positive or a negative answer.

A 3.3.1: B is correct. In fact, it is sometimes the way rare diseases are discovered, through a series of cases. A population-based survey may need to be large to identify cases of a rare disease.

A 3.3.2: All three are possible. But the cluster itself really does not tell you any of these. For the cluster to be of relevance for identifying the cause, the cause must cluster and there must be a short time frame between the cause and the onset of the disease.

A 3.3.3: All three may be correct. A statistician can calculate what the probability of this result by chance alone is. The interpretation is then more problematic.

A 3.4.1: A cross-sectional survey can only measure prevalence, incidence requires a study to follow a population for a period of time. Incidence can only be directly calculated if the denominator, base population, has also been counted.

A 3.4.2: Prevalence is changed by all four of these.

A 3.4.3: The correct answer is C. You must use the number of returned surveys rather than the number sent out originally. So the calculation is

$$\frac{850}{1500} \times 100 = 57\%$$

A 3.4.4: A is correct. It is unlikely that patients are now living for less time than they were, and we already knew that disease X has increased in incidence over 15 years.

A 3.5.1: A is correct. A register may be able to identify cases that can then be measured for risk factors which will allow the collection of relative risk. The prevalence is not directly measured by a register, as the number of deaths, cure and out-migration must be collected for the prevalence to be accessible.

A 3.5.2: The ecological fallacy is a source of bias in studies that compare groups of people rather than individuals. Registers collect incidence data for groups, such as geographically delimited areas and then the incidence may be compared to measured risk factors for that group. The fallacy is in regard to the application of the incidence and risk factor to all of the people, on average. This disregards the fact that the individuals in the groups will possess different risks of disease and different levels of exposure.

A 3.5.3: Using the capture-recapture method we estimate the total number of people with diabetes is:

$$N = \frac{C_1 C_2}{R} = \frac{282 \times 209}{181} = 325.6$$

This means that the estimated number of people with diabetes is 325.

A 3.5.4: One of the main assumptions is that the two 'capture' methods are independent. This is fairly unlikely to be correct as the family doctors will often send people to hospital.

A 3.6.1: D is correct. All of the cases have stomach cancer which is the outcome, whilst the distribution of vegetarianism will be mixed across the two groups.

A 3.6.2: C is correct. The outcome of interest is foot ulcer. Smoking is a risk factor and the case-control study is the design of the study.

A 3.6.3: C is correct. When the odds ratio is below one the risk of the outcome is reduced with an increase in the exposure.

A 3.6.4: B is correct. The odds ratio is calculated from a case-control study, not the risk ratio. Ascertainment of cases may be retrospective, and the ratio of cases to controls may vary.

A 3.6.5: C is not a disadvantage. In fact the case-control study should not be used for common diseases, but for rare ones.

A 3.7.1: C is correct. Cohort studies need to be very large when investigating rare diseases. For this reason case-control studies are more feasible. It is not possible to identify all risk factors for an outcome before conducting a study.

A 3.7.2: D is correct. Loss-to-follow-up is a source of bias and is relevant. However, the reasons for this are varied, and leaving school may make people more difficult to trace, but not impossible.

A 3.7.3: C is correct, the others are RCT (A), case-control (B) and ecological study (D).

A 3.7.4: D is correct. At the start of the cohort study none of the participants should have the outcome, which is asthma. The cohort must have a mixture of bottle and breastfed babies to make the analysis possible.

A 3.8.1: The correct answer is D. Blinding would lead to A, and the randomization will specifically not match patients with treatments.

A 3.8.2: A is the correct answer. B is not incorrect, for example there have been trials of resuscitation techniques following a heart attack. The patient cannot be consented as they will be unconscious. The patients who do not complete the course should remain included in the analysis, known as an intention-to-treat analysis.

A 3.8.3: D is correct. Patients may refuse to be part of an RCT, or they may not be suitable. Many RCTs are not published. Patients may be aware of their allocation, and this relies on the level of blinding imposed on the study.

A 3.8.4: A is correct. There are many RCTs conducted on life-threatening diseases, and they generally will compare the existing treatment with a new one that may be better or worse. An RCT has not been conducted on many interventions that have been used for a long time or which are clearly beneficial.

A 3.8.5: B is correct. It is possible to assess adherence to treatments, for example those that require a patient to attend some form of treatment. The ITT is used as a consequence of people withdrawing from the study.

A 3.9.1: B is correct. As the data is not quantitative, it presents less opportunity for statistical analyses. One of the aims of qualitative research may be to help formulate the research questions. The sampling methods, usually involving choosing participants, make the results less generalizable than methods that use random selection of participants.

A 3.9.2: C is correct.

A 3.9.3: A is False. B is True. C is False. D is False. E is False.

A 3.9.4: A is False. B is False. C is False. D is False. E is True.

A 3.10.1: This is false. The experimental study design, the RCT, allows the researcher to manipulate the exposures that participants experience. This is a stronger design than observing alone.

A 3.10.2: A is correct. Cohort studies are superior to case-control studies as they are generally prospective and less prone to selection bias. An experimental design (RCT) is generally superior to observational study designs.

A 3.10.3: The cohort study is usually a prospective design, in that participants are free from the outcome of interest at the start of the study. And with time the incident cases of disease accrue in the study sample.

A 3.10.4: D is correct. The incidence will give the information for resource allocation for treatment, and the prevalence will aid planning of services. The level of the exposure may be useful for policy and legal challenge. The relative risk will inform the researcher how strong the association between outcome and exposure is.

A 3.10.5: B and D are correct. The design of the RCT has an in-built resistance to confounding bias. But the study design in any specific situation may make either design susceptible to bias. Incidence is directly measured by a cohort study, and this may be used to identify risk factors.

A 3.11.1: C is the correct answer. A systematic review would best describe A. A meta-analysis may only combine results where this is statistically appropriate.

A 3.11.2: This is false. Some publications contain both review and meta-analysis but this is not necessary.

A 3.11.3: A is correct. Systematic reviews may or may not include meta-analysis and these are both used for helping clinicians be more effective. Publication bias is one of the major problems for any study of clinical effectiveness.

A 3.12.1: There is a long list – but here are some highlights:

- Malignant melanoma from sunlight exposure and sunbed use
- Myocardial infarction and cholesterol, hypertension and obesity
- Lung cancer and smoking tobacco
- Lung cancer and radon gas in houses

A 3.12.2: This is an ecological study design, as it compares observations on people and not individuals.

A 4.1.1: The four main types are qualitative nominal, qualitative ordinal, quantitative discrete and quantitative continuous.

A 4.1.2:
A Height is quantitative continuous, as the underlying data is continuous. This remains true even when the data is collected in discrete values, such as in metres or centimetres.
B Sex is qualitative nominal as there is no natural ordering to the categories.
C Number of children is a count, and as such is integer and therefore quantitative discrete.
D Type of degree is nominal, although there may be flexibility in this, as some degrees are 'higher' than others. For example a master's degree follows an undergraduate degree, which would lead to the data being ordinal.
E Marital status is nominal as there is no natural ordering.
F Cancer staging is ordinal, as the categories do not relate to each other in a straightforward numerical sense, but cancer stage 4 has a poorer prognosis than stage 1.

A 4.1.3:
A Weight is a ratio scale.
B Number of moles on a person's skin is a ratio scale.
C Date of a person's birthday is an interval scale.
D Altitude above sea-level is an interval scale.
E Income in dollars is a ratio scale.

A 4.2.1:

A This is a nominal variable, and you would use a pie chart or bar chart to display the count or proportion of people by ethnic group.

B This is a discrete numeric data type, and could be displayed in a histogram. You would need to define the bins in which to place the data.

C This is also a discrete numeric data type, and could be displayed in a histogram. Again, you would need to define the bins in which to place the data.

D This is continuous numeric data, and should be displayed in a histogram, or possibly as a boxplot.

E Here there are two sets of data, and as such could be displayed as a scatterplot. You would probably assign the age as the x-axis, as this is most likely to be the independent variable.

A 4.2.2: True. The vertical axis (y) is usually reserved for the dependent variable.

A 4.2.3: B, E and F are true, although, under certain circumstances the mode and mean will also be represented by the median.

A 4.3.1: The mean is 5.74 (to 2 decimal places) and the median is 4.95. The mode is not really able to be calculated, as all values have a frequency of one.

A 4.3.2: The outlier in the data is the '15.15' data value. If you remove this from the data the mean and the median becomes 4.4. This illustrates how the outlier affects the mean much more than the median.

A 4.3.3: The mean, median and mode are all the same value for the normal distribution. However, the mean is the most usual method for reporting the average for the normal distribution and is explicitly used in its equation.

A 4.3.4: True. As we showed in Q 4.3.2, the mean is affected by outliers.

A 4.3.5: C is correct. The median is based on the 50th percentile.

A 4.4.1: The measures of spread are the range, the standard deviation and the inter-quartile range.

A 4.4.2: The range is 1.1 to 15.15. The standard deviation is 4.39 (to 2 decimal places) and the inter-quartile range is 2.75 to 7.15.

A 4.4.3: The first job is to identify the outlier, which for these data is the value 15.15. Removing this has a large impact on the range, which now becomes 1.1 to 7.7. This is one of the reasons that the range is not used extensively as the measure of spread. The standard deviation has been reduced to 2.38, whilst the inter-quartile range is now 2.2 to 6.6.

A 4.4.4: D is correct. The quartile is the divider of the data, rather than containing the data. In this example this would be the quarter.

A 4.5.1: A, B, C, D and F are correct. Inwards and outwards migration may both affect the prevalence. This is because cases may leave, or arrive, in the population, and they will change the population size. Death will remove people from the population and they may also be cases, and curing the disease will affect prevalence. Births will add to the population. Treatment will not necessarily affect the prevalence, unless it goes on to cure the disease.

A 4.5.2: The choice of the denominator, the population at risk, and numerator is crucial here. You could argue that the correct numerator are the women with existing cervical cancer, and ignore those who have been cured. This means that the prevalence is:

$$P = \frac{47}{2467} = 0.019 \text{ or 2 cases per 100 women.}$$

A 4.5.3: The prevalence will decrease, as the cases in the prevalent pool are removed.

A 4.6.1: Age, sex, ethnic group and geographical region may all be used to define strata. They may all be considered to be some sort of exposure, and so exposure may also be used. The outcome is unlikely to be used as this is the numerator for calculating the rates.

A 4.6.2: A is correct. Directly standardized rates use an external or standard population.

A 4.6.3: Directly standardized rates may be used. But it would be more usual for indirectly standardized rates to be used, especially as it is likely that the number of cases in each sub-area may be small.

A 4.6.4: You must first determine the strata, which in this case are males and females, and the level of reporting of the rate, which we will use per 100 person-years. The rates are:

$$\text{Males: } \frac{28}{2100} \times 100 = 1.33$$

$$\text{Females: } \frac{47}{2398} \times 100 = 1.96$$

A 4.6.5: The overall crude rate is $\frac{28 + 27}{2100 + 2398} \times 100 = 1.22$

A 4.7.1: The relative risk reduction needs the event rates, or rates of the outcome, in the exposed and unexposed groups. These require the measurement of the number of cases and non-cases who are exposed and unexposed to the risk factor under investigation.

A 4.7.2: B and C are correct. A relative risk compares two groups, such as an exposed and an unexposed group. The relative risk reduction also compares two groups, estimating the amount that risk will change between two groups.

A 4.7.3: The relative risk in this case will be described by the risk ratio. For this to be calculated you also need to know the number of people with hypertension who were in the warm houses. This is simply the total number with hypertension (386) minus the number in cold houses (232), which gives 154 cases. The relative risk for the exposed group, which are those in warm houses is

$$EER = \frac{154}{468} = 0.329$$

and the risk for cold houses is

$$UER = \frac{230}{445} = 0.517$$

This leads to a risk ratio of

$$RR = \frac{0.329}{0.517} = 0.637$$

A 4.7.4: This study showed that the risk of hypertension reduced for those living in warm houses. This may be described as being 'protective'. You could go further and say that the risk was reduced by 36.9%.

A 4.8.1: The correct interpretation is that people who ate food from the Bistro had 2.46 times the risk of developing food poisoning compared to people who did not eat food from the Bistro.

A 4.8.2: The odds ratio is not appropriate for common diseases, as the odds ratio becomes more divergent from the risk ratio as the disease becomes more common.

A 4.8.3: You need to know how many controls in total, or at least the number who were not exposed.

A 4.8.4: The odds ratio is:

$$OR = \frac{68/77}{24/121} = 4.45$$

A 4.8.5: The odds ratio is greater than one and therefore we can infer that the exposure is associated with the risk of the disease.

A 4.9.1: This is false, as the standard error is the standard deviation divided by the square root of the number of observations. As the number of observations will always be one or more, then this is false.

A 4.9.2: The z-test requires the mean, standard deviation and the number of observations. The p-value may then be calculated, but is not required to calculate the z-value. The type I error level allows the test to reject, or not, the hypothesis being tested.

A 4.9.3: The z-score of the mean blood pressure for 400 participants requires a standard error which is the standard deviation divided by the square root of the number of observations. The z-score for 400 participants is therefore greater than a z-score where the standard deviation is divided by the square root of 4000. Therefore A is correct.

A 4.10.1: This is a fairly large odds ratio, suggesting that there is an association between the risk of the disease and the exposure being tested. But the confidence interval includes 1, that is the lower bound is less than 1. Therefore this is not statistically significant, and you cannot deduce that the null hypothesis of no association can be rejected.

A 4.10.2: This is false. The 95% confidence interval is narrower than the 99% confidence interval. A simple way to remember this is that the 99% interval is more stringent than the 95% interval, and therefore is more likely to include the null hypothesis.

A 4.10.3: The prevalence of asthma in the practice was:

$$P = \frac{190}{4876} = 0.039$$

which represents 39 persons per 1000 having asthma at that point in time. The standard error of the prevalence is

$$SE = \sqrt{\frac{0.039(1-0.039)}{4876}} = 0.003$$

The upper (*UCI*) and lower (*LCI*) bounds of the confidence interval are, respectively:

$$UCI = 0.039 + (0.05 \times SE) = 0.0392$$

$$\text{and } LCI = 0.039 - (0.05 \times SE) = 0.0388$$

A 4.10.4: B is correct. The values are normally distributed on a log scale and therefore should be used for the calculation of confidence intervals.

A 5.1.1: The three main types of bias are selection, information and confounding.

A 5.1.2: B is the correct answer. Of course, you could also collect the wrong information on the wrong people, which would be information bias, at the same time.

A 5.1.3: A confounder is a cause of the outcome and a cause of the exposure, so this is true.

A 5.1.4: A is correct. Accuracy is a lack of systematic error. A lack of random error is precision.

A 5.2.1: C is correct. Bias can usually be anticipated when a study is being designed. Confounding leads to systematic error.

A 5.2.2: This potentially collects information in an inappropriate way and may lead to information bias.

A 5.2.3: Information bias can be anticipated at the study-design stage and action should be put in place to reduce this to a minimum.

A 5.3.1: C is the correct answer. Random allocation does not mean that the experimenter will not know which arm of a trial the subject has been allocated to. Comparing the sample to a population requires that the original subject selection was done to represent the population. The treatments are assigned specifically so that they disregard the characteristics of the subject.

A 5.3.2: This is true and is often known as participation bias.

A 5.3.3: Selection bias is collecting the right data on the wrong people.

A 5.3.4: Recruiting participants from an occupational setting runs the risk of the healthy worker effect. Losses-to-follow-up may actually be reduced using an occupational setting.

A 5.3.5: Random digit dialling will only contact people who are in their homes when you ring, and who have access to a telephone. Snowballing may lead to a biased sample of those in certain sections of a population. A disease register may offer a very good approach to sampling a population of cases. If you want to sample from a general population, the electoral roll may be most appropriate, as long as you wish to recruit people eligible to vote.

A 5.4.1: A confounder must be a cause of the outcome, so this is true.

A 5.4.2: This is false as a confounder must be associated with the exposure of interest.

A 5.4.3: Confounding is reduced because of the random allocation to groups, so C is correct.

References

Aldrich, T. and Sinks, T. (2002) Things to know and do about cancer clusters. Cancer Investigation 20(5-6), 810–816.

Anscombe, F.J. (1973) Graphs in statistical analysis. The American Statistician 27, 17–21.

Antes, G., Sauerland, S. and Seiler, C.M. (2006) Evidence-based medicine – from best research evidence to a better surgical practice and health care. Langenbecks Archives of Surgery 391, 61–67.

Antman, E.M., Lau, J., Kupelnick, B., Mosteller, F. and Chalmers, T.C. (1992) A comparison of results of meta-analyses of randomized control trials and recommendations of clinical experts. Treatments for myocardial infarction. JAMA 268, 240–248.

Armstrong, D. (2009) Commentary: Indeterminate sick-men – a commentary on Jewson's 'Disappearance of the sick-man from medical cosmology'. International Journal of Epidemiology 38, 642–645.

Aronson, J.K. (2003) Anecdotes as evidence. BMJ 326, 1346.

Ault, K.A., Future II Study Group (2007) Effect of prophylactic human papillomavirus L1 virus-like-particle vaccine on risk of cervical intraepithelial neoplasia grade 2, grade 3, and adenocarcinoma in situ: a combined analysis of four randomised clinical trials. Lancet 369(9576), 1861–1868.

Bampton, P.A., Sandford, J.J. and Young, G.P. (2007) Achieving long-term compliance with colonoscopic surveillance guidelines for patients at increased risk of colorectal cancer in Australia. International Journal of Clinical Practice 61, 510–513.

Becker, H.S., Geer, B., Hughes, E.C. and Strauss, A.L. (1961) Boys in White: Student Culture in Medical School. University of Chicago Press, Chicago.

Belch, J., MacCuish, A., Campbell, I., et al. (2008). The prevention of progression of arterial disease and diabetes (POPADAD) trial: factorial randomised placebo controlled trial of aspirin and antioxidants in patients with diabetes and asymptomatic peripheral arterial disease. BMJ 337, 1840.

Boorstin, D.J. and Waterman, N. (1995) Cleopatra's Nose: Essays on the Unexpected. Blackstone, Ashland.

Breslow, N.E. and Day, N.E. (1980) Statistical Methods in Cancer Research. 1: The Analysis of Case-Control Studies. IARC, Lyon.

Brown, D. (2007) Tricks of the Mind. 4 Books, London.

Brown, P. (1991) Themes in medical sociology. Journal of Health Politics, Policy and Law 16(3), 595–604.

Campbell, D., Green, S., Pitt, V. and Zavarsek, S. (2006) Volume outcome project: hospital or clinician volume or specialisation in cancer care. Available from: http://www.cochrane.org.au/projects/vol_surg.php.

Caracelli, V.J. and Greene, J.C. (1997) Crafting mixed-method evaluation designs. In: Greene, J.C. and Caracelli, V.J. (eds) Advances in Mixed-Method Evaluation: The Challenges and Benefits of Integrating Diverse Paradigms. Jossey-Bass, San Francisco, pp. 19–32.

Davis, D.A., Mazmanian, P.E., Fordis, M., Van Harrison, R., Thorpe, K.E. and Perrier, L. (2006) Accuracy of physician self-assessment compared with observed measures of competence: a systematic review. JAMA 296(9), 1094–1102.

Doll, R. and Hill, A.B. (1950) Smoking and carcinoma of the lung; preliminary report. British Medical Journal 4682, 739–748.

Doll, R. and Hill, A.B. (1954) The mortality of doctors in relation to their smoking habits. British Medical Journal 1(4877), 1451–1455.

Durkheim, E. (1947) The Divison of Labour in Society. The Free Press, Glencoe.

Forbes, S.S., Stephen, W.J., Harper, W.L., et al. (2008) Implementation of evidence-based practices for surgical site infection prophylaxis: results of a pre- and postintervention study. Journal of the American College of Surgeons 207, 336–341.

Foster, N.E., Thomas, E., Barlas, P., Hill, J.C., Young, J., Mason, E. and Hay, E.M. (2007) Acupuncture as an adjunct to exercise based physiotherapy for osteoarthritis of the knee: randomized controlled trial. BMJ 335, 436–440.

Fox, R. (1989) The Sociology of Medicine: A Participant Observer's View. Prentice-Hall, Englewood Cliffs.

Fraumeni, J.F. Jr, Lloyd, J.W., Smith, E.M. and Wagoner, J.K. (1969) Cancer mortality among nuns: role of marital status in etiology of neoplastic disease in women. Journal of the National Cancer Institute 42(3), 455–468.

Galileo (1638) Discorsi e dimostrazioni matematiche. Translation in: Crew, H. and de Salvio, A., translators, [1914] (1954) Dialogues Concerning Two New Sciences. Dover Publications Inc., New York, NY. ISBN 486-60099-8.

Gasparini, R. and Panatto, D. (2009) Cervical cancer: from Hippocrates through Rigoni-Stern to zur Hausen. Vaccine 27 Suppl 1, A4–5.

Graunt, J. (1939) Natural and Political Observations Made Upon the Bills of Mortality. Wilcox, W.F. (ed) Reprint of first edition. The Johns Hopkins Press, Maryland.

Greenland, S. and Robins, J.M. (1986) Identifiability, exchangeability, and epidemiological confounding. International Journal of Epidemiology 15(3), 413–419.

Greenland, S., Pearl, J. and Robins, J.M. (1999) Causal diagrams for epidemiologic research. Epidemiology 10(1), 37–48.

Grol, R. (2001) Successes and failures in the implementation of evidence-based guidelines for clinical practice. Medical Care 39(8), II46–54.

Gross, P.R. and Levitt, N. (1998) Higher Superstition: The Academic Left and Its Quarrels With Science. Johns Hopkins University Press, London.

Hardman, J. and Carlson, G.L. (2008) Evidence-based perioperative care is lost in translation. British Journal of Surgery 9, 807–808.

Hartge, P. (1999) Raising response rates: Getting to yes. Epidemiology 10, 105–107.

Henderson, M. and Page, L. (2007) Appraising the evidence: what is selection bias? Evidence-Based Mental Health 10(3), 67–68.

Hernan, M.A., Hernandez-Diaz, S. and Robins, J.M. (2004) A structural approach to selection bias. Epidemiology 15(5), 615–625.

Hill, A.B. (1965) The environment and disease: association or causation? Proceedings of the Royal Society of Medicine 58, 295–300.

Holt, V.L., Daling, J.R., Stergachis, A., Voigt, L.F. and Weiss, N.S. (1991) Results and effect of refusal recontact in a case-control study of ectopic pregnancy. Epidemiology 2, 375–379.

Howes, N., Chagla, L., Thorpe, M. and McCulloch, P. (1997) Surgical practice is evidence based. British Journal of Surgery 84, 1220–1223.

Hyde, L. (1999) Trickster Makes This World: Mischief, Myth, and Art. North Point Press, New York.

Jewson, N.D. (2009) The disappearance of the sick-man from medical cosmology, 1770–1870. International Journal of Epidemiology 38(3), 622–633.

Keating, N.L., Beth Landrum, M., Arora, N.K., Malin, J.L., Ganz, P.A., van Ryn, M. and Weeks, J.C. (2010) Cancer patients' roles in treatment decisions: do characteristics of the decision influence roles? Journal of Clinical Oncology 28(28), 4364–4370.

Kelly, M.J., Lloyd, T.D., Marshall, D., Garcea, G., Sutton, C.D. and Beach, M. (2003) A snapshot of MDT working and patient mapping in the UK colorectal cancer centres in 2002. Colorectal Disease 5(6), 577–581.

Kilbourne, E. (1973) The molecular epidemiology of influenza. The Journal of Infectious Diseases 127(4), 478–487.

Kwon, H.L., Ortiz, B., Swaner, R., Shoemaker, K., Jean-Louis, B., Northridge, M.E., Vaughan, R.D., Marx, T., Goodman, A., Borrell, L.N. and Nicholas, S.W. (2006) Childhood asthma and extreme values of body mass index: the Harlem Children's Zone Asthma Initiative. Journal of Urban Health 83(3), 421–433.

Lamberts, H., Wood, M. and Hofmans-Okkes, I. (1993) The International Classification of Primary Care in the European Community. Oxford University Press, Oxford.

Lassen, K., Hannemann, P., Ljungqvist, O., et al. (2005) Patterns in current perioperative practice: survey of colorectal surgeons in five northern European countries. BMJ 330, 1420–1421.

Last, J.M. (2000) A Dictionary of Epidemiology. Oxford University Press, New York.

Law, G.R., Smith, A.G., Roman, E. and United Kingdom Childhood Cancer Study Investigators (2002) The importance of full participation: lessons from a national case-control study. BJC 86(3), 350–355.

Law, G.R., Parslow, R.C., Roman, E. and United Kingdom Childhood Cancer Study Investigators (2003) Childhood cancer and population mixing. American Journal of Epidemiology 158(4), 328–336.

Lorenz, K. (1966) On Aggression, trans. M. Latzke. Routledge, London.

Madigan, M.P., Troisi, R., Potischman, N., et al. (2000) Characteristics of respondents and non-respondents from a case-control study of breast cancer in younger women. International Journal of Epidemiology 29, 793–798.

Marx, M.H. (1963) Theories in Contemporary Psychology. Macmillan, New York.

McGlynn, E.A., Asch S.M., Adams J., et al. (2003) The quality of health care delivered to adults in the United States. NEJM 348, 2635–2645.

McNamee, R. (2003) Confounding and confounders. Occupational and Environmental Medicine 60(3), 227–234.

Medical Research Council (1948) Streptomycin treatment of pulmonary tuberculosis. British Medical Journal 2(4582), 769–782.

Merton, R.K., Reader, G.G. and Kendall, P.L. (eds) (1957) The Student-Physician: Introductory Studies in the Sociology of Medical Education. Harvard University Press, Cambridge.

Moerman, D.E. and Jonas, W.B. (2002) Deconstructing the placebo effect and finding the meaning response. Annals of Internal Medicine 136(6), 471–476.

Müller-Lyer, F.C. (1886) Zur Lehre von den optischen Tauschungen über Kontrast und Konfluxion. Zeitschr Psychol 10, 421–431.

Norton, J.D. (2005) What is Einstein's legacy to me? Imagine 13(1).

Park, R. (1927) Quoted in http://www.newworldencyclopedia.org/entry/Robert_E._Park, retrieved 03/05/2012.

Parsons, T. (1951) The Social System. The Free Press, Glencoe.

Pearl, J. (2000) Causality: Models, Reasoning and Inference. Cambridge University Press, Cambridge.

Rescher, N. (1979) The ontology of the possible. In: Loux, M.J. (ed) The Possible and the Actual: Readings in the Metaphysics of Modality. Cornell University Press, New York.

Robison, L.L. and Daigle, A. (1984) Control selection using random digit dialling for cases of childhood cancer. American Journal of Epidemiology 120, 164–166.

Rossman, G.B. and Wilson, B.L. (1985) Numbers and words: Combining quantitative and qualitative methods in a single large-scale evaluation study. Evaluation Review 9(5), 627–643.

Rossman, G.B. and Wilson, B.L. (1994) Numbers and words revisited: being 'shamelessly eclectic'. Quality and Quantity 28, 315–327.

Roth, P. (2004) The Plot Against America. Houghton Mifflin.

Rothman, K.J. (1976) Causes. American Journal of Epidemiology 104(6), 587–592.

Rothman, K.J. (1990) A sobering start for the cluster busters' conference. American Journal of Epidemiology 132(1 Suppl), S6-13.

Rothman, K.J. and Greenland, S. (1998) Modern Epidemiology. Lippincott Williams & Wilkins, Baltimore, USA.

Rubin, S.C. (2001) Cervical cancer: successes and failures. CA: A Cancer Journal for Clinicians 51(2), 89–91.

Rutan, B. (2004) Black Sky: The Race for Space. Discovery Channel USA, release date 2004.

Sackett, D.L., Rosenberg, W.M., Gray, J.A., Haynes, R.B. and Richardson, W.S. (1996) Evidence based medicine: what it is and what it isn't. BMJ 312(7023), 71–72.

Sargent, R.P., Shepard, R.M. and Glantz, S.A. (2004) Reduced incidence of admissions for myocardial infarction associated with public smoking ban: before and after study. BMJ 328, 977–978.

Schlesselman, J.J. and Stolley, P.D. (1982) Case-Control Studies: Design, Conduct, Analysis. Oxford University Press.

Skrabanek, P. (1988) Cervical cancer in nuns and prostitutes: A plea for scientific continence. Journal of Clinical Epidemiology 41, 577–582.

Slattery, M., Overall, J., Abbott, T., French, T., Robinson, L. and Gardner, J. (1989) Sexual activity, contraception, genital infections, and cervical cancer: Support for a sexually transmitted disease hypothesis. American Journal of Epidemiology 130, 248–258.

Slim, K. (2005) Limits of evidence-based surgery. World Journal of Surgery 29, 606–609.

Slim, K., Panis, Y. and Chipponi, J. (2004) Half of the currecnt practice of gastrointestinal surgery is against the evidence: a survery of the French Society of Digestive Surgery. Journal of Gastrointestinal Surgery 8, 1079–1082.

Smith, G.C. and Pell, J.P. (2003) Parachute use to prevent death and major trauma related to gravitational challenge: systematic review of randomised controlled trials. BMJ 327(7429), 1459–1461.

Social Exclusion Task Force (2008) Reaching Out: Think Family. Analysis and Themes from the Families At Risk Review. Social Exclusion Task Force, Cabinet Office, London.

Solomon, M.J. and McLeod, R.S. (1995) Should we be performing more randomized controlled trials evaluating surgical operations? Surgery 118, 459–467.

Steinberg, K.K., Relling, M.V., Gallagher, M.L., et al. (2007) Genetic studies of a cluster of acute lymphoblastic leukemia cases in Churchill County, Nevada. Environmental Health Perspectives 115, 158–164.

Studdert, D.M., Mello, M.M., Gawande, A.A., Gandhi, T.K., Kachalia, A., Yoon, C., Puopolo, A.L. and Brennan, T.A. (2006) Claims, errors, and compensation payments in medical malpractice litigation. NEJM 354(19), 2024–2033.

Thom, D.H., Kravitz, R.L., Kelly-Rief, S., Sprinkle, R.V., Hopkins, J.R. and Rubenstein, L.V. (2004) A new instrument to measure appropriateness of services in primary care. International Journal for Quality in Health Care 16(2), 133–140.

Tu, Y.-K., West, R.W., Ellison, G.D.H. and Gilthorpe, M.S. (2004) Why evidence for the fetal origins of adult disease can be statistical artifact: the reversal paradox examined for hypertension. American Journal of Epidemiology 161(1), 27–32.

UKCCS Investigators (2000) The United Kingdom Childhood Cancer Study: objectives, materials and methods. BJC 82, 1073–1102.

Verdecchia, A., Micheli, A., Colonna, M., Moreno, V., Izarzugaza, M.I., Paci, E. and the Europreval Working Group (2002) A comparative analysis of cancer prevalence in cancer registry areas of France, Italy and Spain. Annals of Oncology 13, 1128–1139.

Wacholder, S., McLaughlin, J.K., Silverman, D.T. and Mandel, J.S. (1992a) Selection of controls in case-control studies. I. Principles. American Journal of Epidemiology 135(9), 1019–1028.

Wacholder, S., Silverman, D.T., McLaughlin, J.K. and Mandel, S. (1992b) Selection of controls in case-control studies. II. Types of controls. American Journal of Epidemiology 135(9), 1029–1041.

Wakefield, A.J., Murch, S.H., Anthony, A., et al. (1998) Ileal-lymphoid-nodular hyperplasia, non-specific colitis, and pervasive developmental disorder in children. Lancet 351, 637–641.

Watkins, S.J. (2000) Doctors and lawyers should get probability theory right. BMJ 320, 2.

Weed, L.L. (1969) Medical Records, Medical Education, and Patient Care. The Press of Case Western Reserve University, Cleveland.

Weinberg, C.R. (2005) Barker meets Simpson. American Journal of Epidemiology 161(1), 33–35.

Westergren, A., Karlsson, S., Andersson, P., Ohlsson, O. and Hallberg, I.R. (2001) Eating difficulties, need for assisted eating, nutritional status and pressure ulcers in patients admitted for stroke rehabilitation. Journal of Clinical Nursing 10, 257–269.

WHO (1948) Preamble to the Constitution of the World Health Organization as Adopted by the International Health Conference. WHO, New York.

WHO (2006) Cancer. Fact Sheets 297. Retrieved 15/3/2007, from http://www.who.int/mediacentre/factsheets/fs297/en/index.html.

Willis, J. (1979) Lecture Notes on Psychiatry. Blackwell Scientific Publications, Oxford.

Wootton, D. (2006) Bad Medicine: Doctors Doing Harm Since Hippocrates. OUP, Oxford.

Wrensch, M., Mike, R., Lee, M. and Neuhaus, J. (2000) Are prior head injuries or diagnostic X-rays associated with glioma in adults? The effects of control selection bias. Neuroepidemiology 19, 234–244.

Wyatt, J.C. (1995) Hospital information management: the need for clinical leadership. British Medical Journal 311, 175–178.

Young, J.M., Hollands, M.J. and Solomon, M.J. (2006) Surgeons' participation in continuing medical education: is it evidence-based? Medical Education 40(5), 423–429.

Youngson, R. (1992) Dictionary of Medicine. Harper Collins, Glasgow.

Index

Absolute risk reduction (ARR), 154
Anecdote
    Bolam test, 58
    in clinical medicine, 55–56
    controversy, 57
    description, 54–55
    in epidemiology, 56
    problems, 57–58
    research hypotheses, 57
    self-test questions and answers, 58, 201
    strengths and weaknesses, 58
    usage in science, 55
ARR. *See* Absolute risk reduction (ARR)

Bias
    definitions, 177
    information, 181
    non-random allocation methods, 177
    sampling error, 177
    selection, 177–180
    self-test questions and answers, 182, 208
    types, 177

Case-control study
    case selection, 77
    characteristics, 76
    clinician's approach, 75
    control selection, 77–79
    counterfactual population, 76
    description, 75
    exposure time frames, 79
    matching, 79
    odds ratio, 81
    participation, 79–80
    participation effects, 80–81
    'rare disease' assumption, 77
    self-test questions and answers, 83, 202
    strengths and weaknesses, 81–82
Causation
    component model, 45–46

concept, inference, 39
    counterfactual approach, 38
    counterfactual world, 44
    DAGs, 46
    disease aetiology, 37
    Hill's roadmap, 44–45
    induction and latent periods, 40–41
    infectious pathogens, 46
    initiator and promoter, 41
    Koch's postulates, 43
    light bulb analogy, 39
    meta-analysis, 44
    paths link variables, 48
    philosophical musings, 36–37
    RCTs, 44
    representation, outcome, 39
    self-test questions and answers, 41–42,
        46–47, 51, 200–201
    strength, effect, 40
    study designs, 38
    types, 38
Cochrane Collaboration, 115, 116
Cohort study
    anatomy, 84–85
    British Births Survey (BBS), 88
    The British Doctors' study, 87–88
    and case-control study, 88
    choosing members, 85
    description, 83
    The Framingham Heart Study, 88
    household panel surveys, 88–89
    loss-to-follow-up, 89
    prospective or retrospective, 86
    risk ratio, 87
    self-test questions and answers, 90–91,
        202–203
    strengths and weaknesses, 89
    types, 85–86
    unfeasible cohort, 90
Confounding
    analysis phase, 196
    causal pathways, 197

Confounding (*continued*)
  DAGs, 195
  definition, 193–194
  lung cancer, 194
  objective method, 194–195
  RCT, 196
  self-test questions and answers,
      197–198, 209
  statistical computer packages, 197
Cross-sectional survey
  anatomy, 65
  census, 66
  disease prevalence, 65–66
  longitudinal studies, 66
  metaphor, 64–65
  prevalence studies for causation, 66
  self-test questions and answers, 67–68,
      201–202
  strengths and weaknesses, 67

DAGs. *See* Directed acyclic graphs (DAGs)
Data presentation
  ABO blood group data, bar chart, 126
  agreeable disagreeableness, 124
  Anscombe's quartet, 130, 131
  box-and-whisker plot, 128–129
  continuous/discrete, 123
  defining scales, 123
  epidemiological research, 123
  frequency table, 125–126
  histograms
      age, 127
      birth weight data in kg, 127, 128
  nominal/ordinal, 122–123
  pie chart, ABO blood group data, 126
  qualitative/quantitative, variables,
      121–122
  scatterplots, 129
  self-test questions and answers, 124–125,
      130, 204, 205
Directed acyclic graphs (DAGs)
  causal relationships, system, 48
  confounding variable, 197
  epidemiological analyses, data, 51
  hypothetical, 196
  lung cancer, 47, 195
  nodes and arcs, 48–50
  speculative nature, 50
  strengths and weaknesses, 50
Disease registers
  anatomy, 68–69

applications, 70
assigning subgroup, 72–73
cases identification, sources, 69
causality, 72
ecological fallacy, 74
ecological techniques, 70–71
incidence, 68, 72
issues of consent, 70
self-test questions and answers,
    75, 202
strengths and weaknesses, 73–74

EBM. *See* Evidence-based medicine (EBM)
EBP. *See* Evidence-based practice (EBP)
Epidemiologist's toolkit
  Anecdote, 54–59, 118
  case-control study, 75–83
  cases
      case report, in disease
          recognition, 60–61
      case series, systematic collection
          of reports, 61–62
      clusters, 62–63
  cohort study, 83–91
  cross-sectional survey, 64–68
  diagnosis process, 53
  disease registers, 68–75
  hierarchy of evidence, 108–113
  HPV discovery, 118–119
  preventative vaccines, 119
  progress in early detection, 53
  qualitative research, 102–108
  RCT, 91–102
  screening process, 53
  study designs, 52
  systematic review and meta-analysis,
      113–117
  treatments, 53–54
Errors
  contrasting accuracy and
      precision, 176
  counterfactual approach,
      causation, 175
  definitions, 173
  development, theories, 173
  external validity, 177
  potential sources, 175
  science and nature, 174
  spotting error, 174–175
  statistical techniques, 175
Evidence-based medicine (EBM), 16

Evidence-based practice (EBP)
    diagnosis and treatment decisions, 16
    EBM, 16
    statistical methods, 17

Grounded theory (GT), 105
GT. *See* Grounded theory (GT)

Hierarchy of evidence
    evidence-based medicine, 108
    healthcare, 109
    limitations, 111
    official agencies, 111–112
    practitioner's approach, 108–109
    self-test questions and answers, 112–113,
        203–204
    systematic approach, 109–110
Hormone replacement therapy
        (HRT), 10
HRT. *See* Hormone replacement therapy
        (HRT)
Hypotheses
    aligned statistical practice, 10
    falsifiable, 9
    HRT, 10
    null hypothesis, 10
    Occam's razor, 10
Hypothesis testing
    definition, 165–166
    interpretation, p-value, 167
    probability, measure, 164–165
    self-test questions and answers,
        168, 207
    shapes, distributions, 167
    standard normal, 165
    statistical distributions, smooth curves,
        163–164
    statistical testing, p-value, 166–167
    z-test, 167, 168

Information bias
    diagnosis, 186
    disease status, participants, 186
    epidemiology studies, 184
    life events, 187
    medical record, 187
    misclassification
        differential, 187
        non-differential, 187

self-test questions and answers,
        188, 208
    surrogate sources, data, 186
    trained and monitored,
        interviewers, 185
Inter-quartile range (IQR)
    continuous and discrete metric
        variables, 138
    median value, 137
IQR. *See* Inter-quartile range (IQR)

Measures of location
    data types, 132
    distribution, measurements, 135
    extreme values, outliers, 134
    Gaussian distribution/
        bell-curve curve, 133
    median, 133–134
    mode, 134
    self-test questions and answers,
        139, 205
    statistical approach, 131
    weighted means, 132
Medical sociology
    control, uncertainty, 32–33
    individuals and populations, 31
    measurement and communication
        consultation mapping
            approach, 33
        illness, 33
        pathology, 34
        shared-decision making, 35
        social constructs, 35
    measurement, ideas, 30
    national/regional issue, 30
    self-test questions and answers,
        35, 200
    sick role, 31–32

Non-random methods
    accidental or haphazard sampling, 22
    purposive, purposeful or judgemental
        sampling, 22
    snowball sampling, 22
Numbers
    absolute and relative risks, 154
    anaesthesiology, 155–156
    AR, 151–152
    centralization, services, 155
    communication, 156

Numbers (*continued*)
    confidence intervals
        interpretation, 170
        log scale, 171
        null hypothesis, 172
        odds ratio, rate ratio, 172
        percentage, 169–170
        prevalence, 170–171
        p-value, 169
        student's t-distribution, 170
    data presentation, 125–130
    hypothesis testing, 163–168
    incidence, disease
        bath analogy, 143
        cumulative and stratum-specific
            incidence, 148–149
        fatality and mortality, 144–145
        indirectly standardized ratio,
            147–148
        per person per unit time, 144
        person-years, population, 144
        standardization, subgroups, 145
        standard populations, 146, 147
    language, 150
    measures, spread
        boxplot, 139
        IQR, 137–139
        SD, 136–137
    multi-dimensional risk, 157
    odds and odds ratios, 158–163
    prevalence, disease
        bath analogy, 140
        incidence, cure, migration, 141
        point, period or lifetime, 141
        proportion, population, 140–141
        service planning and cause, 140
    self-test questions and answers, 135,
        139, 142–143, 149–150,
        158, 172, 205–208
    types, data, 121–125

Observational and experimental studies
    cholera minimization, 28–29
    field experiments, 28
    laboratory-based experimental
        science, 26
    natural experiments, 26
    probabilistic equivalency, 28
    scientific method framework, 25
    self-test questions and answers, 29, 200
    thought experiments, 26–27

Odds ratios (OR)
    case-control study, 158–159
    odds and probability, 161, 162
    RR, 159–160
    self-test questions and answers,
        162–163, 207
    stroke rehabilitation, 160

Population
    definition, 19
    denominator, 19–20
    progress, sampling, 20

Qualitative research
    constant comparison, 106
    data, 104–105
    description, 103
    grounded theory (GT), 105
    mixed methods, 106–107
    self-test questions and answers,
        107–108, 203

Randomized controlled trials (RCT)
    analysis
        intention to treat, 98–99
        relative risk, 97–98
    anatomy, 92–93
    blinding, 96–97
    categorization, 95
    conduct and reporting, 99–100
    description, 91–92
    drug trials, 100
    experiment use, 93–94
    intervention, 92
    number of people, treatment, 99
    placebo, 96
    self-test questions and answers,
        102, 203
    strengths, 94–95
    strengths and weaknesses,
        100–101
Random methods, sampling
    cluster, 23
    simple probability, 22
    stratified random, 23
    systematic probability, 22–23
RCT. *See* Randomized controlled
    trials (RCT)
Relative risk reduction (RRR), 154

Sampling methods
cluster randomized sampling, 24
HPV, 23
non-random, 21–22
random, 22–23
sample size, 24
SARS. *See* Severe acute respiratory
syndrome (SARS)
Scientific methods
decision making, 14
definition, 7
development, knowledge, 8
epidemiological research, 8
everyday versus scientific
approaches, 11
human senses/instruments, 8
hypotheses, 9–10
Müller-Lyer illusion, 11
observation and measurement, 12
scientific method, 8–9
self-test questions and answers,
14, 199
statistics, 13
theory, 9
trickster attitude, 12
validity and reliability,
measurements, 12
SD. *See* Standard deviation (SD)
Selection bias
exploring non-participation, 191
healthy worker effect, 190
participants, 190–191
population, defined, 188–189
practical and ethical constraints, 191
random sampling strategy, 189–190
regression model, 192
self-test questions and answers,
192–193, 208–209
Severe acute respiratory syndrome
(SARS), 3
SIR. *See* Standardized incidence ratio (SIR)

Standard deviation (SD)
calorie intake, 136–137
measure, spread, 136
quantitative data, 136
Standardized incidence ratio
(SIR), 148
Statistical epidemiology
causes, society, 2–3
Chinese medicine, 3
designs, 23
EBP, 16–17
healthcare professionals, 16
health delivery, 5
measurement, distribution, 1–2
medical sociology, 30–35
non-random methods, 21–22
observational and experimental
studies, 25–29
observation, medical science, 4
power analysis, 23
random methods, 22–23
scientific methods, 7–14
self-test questions and answers, 6–7,
19, 25, 199–200
smoking and lung cancer, 18
sub-disciplines, 6
Systematic review
Cochrane Collaboration, 115
defining the question, 114
and meta-analysis, 113–114,
115–116
review assessment, 115
self-test questions and answers,
117, 204

The British Doctors' study, 87–88
The Framingham Heart Study, 88

z-test, 167, 168